Exercise and Immunology

Current Issues in Exercise Science
Monograph Number 2

Laurel T. Mackinnon, PhD
University of Queensland, Australia

Human Kinetics Books
Champaign, Illinois

Library of Congress Cataloging-in-Publication Data

Mackinnon, Laurel T., 1953-
  Exercise and immunology / Laurel T. Mackinnon
    p.   cm. -- (Current issues in exercise science series, ISSN
  1055-1352 ; monograph, no. 2)
  Includes bibliographical references and index.
  ISBN 0-87322-347-0
  1. Exercise--Immunological aspects. I. Title. II. Series.
QP301.M16   1992
616.07'9--dc20   91-42289
                                                                      CIP

ISBN: 0-87322-347-0

ISSN: 1055-1352

Copyright © 1992 by Laurel T. Mackinnon

Managing Editor and Proofreader: Julia Anderson
Assistant Editors: Laura Bofinger, Kari Nelson, and Elizabeth Bridgett
Copyeditor: Molly Bentsen
Indexer: Sheila Ary
Production Director: Ernie Noa
Typesetting and Text Layout: Angela K. Snyder
Text Design: Keith Blomberg
Cover Design: Hunter Graphics
Printer: United Graphics

Printed in the United States of America

10 9 8 7 6 5 4 3 2 1

Human Kinetics Books
A Division of Human Kinetics Publishers, Inc.
Box 5076, Champaign, IL 61825-5076
1-800-747-4457

Canada Office:
Human Kinetics Publishers, Inc.
P.O. Box 2503, Windsor, ON N8Y 4S2
1-800-465-7301 (in Canada only)

Europe Office:
Human Kinetics Publishers (Europe) Ltd.
P.O. Box IW14
Leeds LS16 6TR
England
0532-781708

Australia Office:
Human Kinetics Publishers (Australia)
P.O. Box 80
Kingswood, SA 5062
(08) 374 0433

To Ian and Scott

Contents

Preface

The rapidly expanding field of exercise and immunology has recently attracted interest from researchers in exercise science, medicine, immunology, physiology, and behavioral science. Interest in the immune response to exercise has arisen for many reasons. First, athletes, coaches, and team physicians want to keep athletes healthy during training and competition. Most elite athletes and their coaches believe that athletes are more susceptible to illness, especially upper respiratory illness, during intense training and major competition. Some illnesses affect the athlete's ability to train and compete, and continued training or competition during illness may be detrimental to the athlete's health.

The attention to exercise and immunity is also shaped by community interest in health promotion. Regular moderate exercise appears to be important in the prevention and treatment of a variety of diseases, including heart disease, obesity, non-insulin-dependent diabetes, hypertension, and osteoporosis. Researchers are now focusing on other diseases with significant lifestyle-associated risk factors, such as cancer, and there is evidence to suggest that people who exercise regularly exhibit lower incidences of certain cancers.

Exercise has come to be prescribed as adjunct therapy for certain diseases, including cancer and acquired immune deficiency syndrome (AIDS). It is used mainly to counteract the physically debilitating effects of the illness and treatment or to improve the patient's physical or psychological state. Because the immune system is intimately involved in cancer and AIDS, scientists are studying the immune response to exercise to determine its effects on disease progress.

Finally, there is a developing interest in exercise and immunology in terms of "psychoneuroimmunology" or "behavioral immunology." Recent studies have shown significant interaction between the neuroendocrine and immune systems. Stress has long been identified as a modulator of immune function. Exercise can be considered a form of physical stress, because many of the hormones capable of immunomodulation also increase during exercise. Exercise appears to be one of several lifestyle factors, such as psychological stress, nutrition, sleep deprivation, and injury, that influence the immune system. Exercise may provide a unique model to study adaptation to stress because many hormonal and physiological responses to exercise change after training.

This monograph is an introduction to the growing field of exercise and immunology. I begin by considering whether athletes are more susceptible to illness than the general population and then review the literature on the effects of exercise on resistance to infectious disease. In chapter 2 I discuss immune function in a brief and cursory overview of an exceedingly complex system. I have deliberately limited the scope of this section, intending only to introduce the nonimmunologist to relevant terminology and concepts. The interested reader may wish to consult an immunology text for more detail.

Chapters 3 through 7 address the effects of exercise on different aspects of immunity, and chapter 8 focuses on clinical implications of exercise for immune function. Finally, I conclude with a model of how exercise may influence immune function and suggest future directions for research.

There is much about exercise and immunology that we do not know, for study is in its infancy. Future research will enhance our understanding of both immune regulation and adaptations to exercise.

Acknowledgments

There are many people to thank for their support over the years and in the writing of this book: Dr. Thomas B. Tomasi, who sparked my initial interest in exercise and immunology; Professor Greg Seymour, for the past few years of fruitful collaboration and many helpful discussions about this book; Dr. Ian Mackinnon, for his critical review of the manuscript and his continued support in all my endeavors; Kate Dwan, for her exhaustive library research; the graduate students who survived my preoccupation with this book; and, finally, the editors of Human Kinetics Publishers, for their support in the book's production.

Chapter 1

Exercise and Resistance to Infectious Illness

Physical fatigue, whether caused by exercise or manual work, has long been considered a factor affecting susceptibility to illness. There is a perception among elite athletes, coaches, and sport physicians that athletes are more susceptible to certain illnesses during intense training and major competition. At the same time, there is common belief that those who exercise regularly are less susceptible to certain illnesses, such as the common cold. But neither perception has been well documented, although the few published studies tend to support a dual effect of exercise (i.e., intense exercise increases susceptibility, and moderate exercise reduces susceptibility) on resistance to illness.

Are Athletes Susceptible to Illness?

A relationship between intense exercise and susceptibility to illness was noted early in this century. Cowles (1918) reported that virtually all cases of pneumonia at a boys' school occurred in athletes and that respiratory infections seemed to progress toward pneumonia after intense exercise and competitive sport. Thirty years later the severity of acute poliomyelitis was found to be related to intense physical activity at a critical time of infection (Horstmann, 1950).

Some athletes appear to suffer high rates of certain illnesses, such as infectious mononucleosis (Foster et al., 1982) and upper respiratory illness (Berglund & Hemmingsson, 1990; Douglas & Hanson, 1978; Peters & Bateman, 1983; Tomasi, Trudeau, Czerwinski, & Erredge, 1982). Frequent illness has also been observed in athletes experiencing "overtraining," a condition characterized by prolonged fatigue and due primarily to excessive training. Much of the evidence is anecdotal, but the few attempts to quantify rates of illness tend to support high incidence, at least among endurance athletes (e.g., distance runners and cross-country skiers). Upper respiratory illness appears to be the most common illness in athletes (Berglund & Hemmingsson).

Athletes also appear more likely to perceive illness and to seek medical care for it than nonathletes (Douglas & Hanson, 1978), possibly because even minor illness may affect normal function (training). However, although there is a general perception that athletes are more susceptible to infectious mononucleosis, nearly 90% of Americans exhibit antibodies to its causal agent, the Epstein-Barr virus, by age 30 (Eichner, 1987a), indicating a high incidence of infection among all young people.

Illness After Intense Endurance Exercise

In an epidemiological study, Peters and Bateman (1983) surveyed 140 runners before and after a 56-km ultramarathon, asking specifically about symptoms of upper respiratory illness (URI; e.g., sore throat, runny nose, cough). Each runner had as a control subject an age-matched nonrunner living in the same household. During the two weeks following the race, 33% of all runners exhibited symptoms of URI, compared to 15% of control subjects. Moreover, there was a graded response—the incidence of illness increased as race time decreased, with nearly half of the fastest runners experiencing illness after the race (Figure 1.1).

These data were supported by a later epidemiological study of nearly 5,000 participants in the 1987 Los Angeles Marathon (Nieman, Johanssen, Lee, & Arabatzis, 1990). Participants who trained more than 97 km a week were twice as likely to exhibit infectious illness (e.g., cold, flu, sore throat) during the 2 months prior to the race as runners who averaged less than 32 km per week (confounding variables such as age, perceived stress levels, and illness in the home were adjusted in the statistical analyses). Moreover, participants in the marathon were more than 5 times more likely to exhibit illness after the race than similarly trained runners who did not compete.

Taken together, the studies by Nieman et al. (1990) and Peters and Bateman (1983) suggest that, in runners, the incidence of infectious illness increases with training volume and after major competition; it is also likely that training volume and competition exert a combined effect on susceptibility to illness.

Illness After Less Intense Exercise

In contrast to the high rates of URI among elite and ultraendurance athletes, the incidence of illness may not be altered by participation in shorter and less competitive events (Nieman, Johanssen, & Lee, 1989). For example, in a random survey of 294 runners in "fun

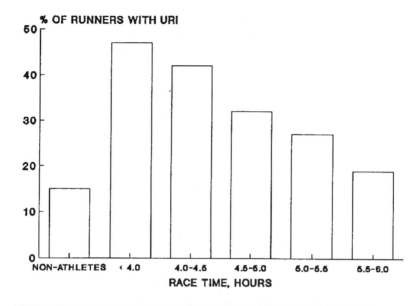

Figure 1.1   Percentages of runners with URI after an ultramarathon. Data represent the percentages of runners and control subjects reporting symptoms of URI during the 2 weeks following a 56-km ultramarathon; runners are grouped by finishing time. Control subjects were age-matched nonathletes living in the same household as the runners. The number of runners exhibiting symptoms of URI was significantly correlated ($r = .995$, $p < .01$) with race time.

Note. This article has been reprinted from the *South African Medical Journal*, Vol. **64**, dated 1 October 1983. "Ultramarathon Running and Upper Respiratory Tract Infections" by E.M. Peters and E.D. Bateman, p. 583. Copyright 1983 by the Medical Association of South Africa. Adapted by permission.

runs" and 5-, 10-, and 21-km races, 30% reported infectious episodes, mainly URI, during the 2 months before the races. However, the incidence of illness was similar during the week before and after the race, suggesting no short-term effect of the races on illness. Incidence was related more to illness in the home than to training volume or distance. Moreover, there was a nonsignificant trend toward lower rates of illness before the race among runners in 21-km races than among those in the shorter runs (23% vs. 31%).

Taken together, then, these studies on URI among athletes suggest that top competitive athletes, and those who engage in very long or intense exercise (e.g., ultramarathon), are more susceptible to URI. In contrast, less competitive athletes, and those engaging in less strenuous exercise, are not more susceptible to URI than the general population. There are limitations, however, to these studies: Illness was documented by self-report, and medical diagnosis was not used to distinguish infectious from noninfectious illnesses (e.g., URI vs. allergy).

Mechanisms Responsible for Upper Respiratory Illness

The mechanisms responsible for the seemingly high incidence of URI among top athletes are not known. It has been suggested that high ventilatory flow rates during prolonged exercise may adversely affect the mucosal surfaces of the upper respiratory tract (Peters & Bateman, 1983; Tomasi et al., 1982). Aspects of nonspecific immunity (an important defense early in infection; see chapter 2) may also be affected by exercise. Recently attention has also been focused on exercise-induced changes in antibody levels in mucosal fluids (discussed in chapter 5).

Resistance to Experimentally Induced Infectious Illness

Epidemiological data on the incidence of illness among athletes are not easily obtained and do not always provide information on resistance to specific illnesses. It is also difficult to quantify or control the level of exercise. Hence, many studies have taken an experimental approach to the question of whether exercise influences resistance to infectious illness. Experimental work on immune reactivity in humans has obvious ethical limitations, and much of the experimental work has been performed on laboratory animals. But most studies using animal models of exercise include forced activity, either swimming or treadmill running, which may induce a stress response that affects immune function.

The earliest work on exercise and immune function focused on the effects of physical fatigue on resistance to infectious illnesses, such as pneumonia and influenza, that were major killers in Western countries before modern antibiotics (Bailey, 1925; Nicholls & Spaeth, 1922; Oppenheimer & Spaeth, 1922). These studies suggested that exercise training prior to infection enhanced resistance, whereas exercise at the time of infection reduced it.

Later studies on the effects of exercise on experimentally induced poliomyelitis followed clinical observations that paralysis was often preceded by intense physical activity at the time of infection (Horstmann, 1950). For example, monkeys (Levinson, Milzer, & Lewin,

1945) and mice (Rosenbaum & Harford, 1953) forced to exercise to exhaustion at the time of poliomyelitis infection exhibited reduced survival rates and increased severity of illness.

Intense exercise also appears to influence resistance to other experimentally induced viral illnesses, such as coxsackievirus and influenza in mice (Cabinian et al., 1990; Ilback, Friman, Beisel, Johnson, & Berendt, 1984; Ilback, Fohlman, & Friman, 1989; Kiel, Smith, Chason, Khatib, & Reyes, 1989; Reyes & Lerner, 1976; Woodruff, 1980). For example, forced swimming during the early stages of viral infection has been shown to increase mortality (Cabinian et al.; Kiel et al.; Ilback et al., 1984), the number of viruses in serum and the heart, and the extent of myocardial lesions in exercised compared with nonexercised animals (Gatmaitin, Chason, & Lerner, 1970; Kiel et al.; Ilback et al., 1989; Reyes & Lerner). Exercised animals also had fewer antibodies to the virus in the blood and a delayed response in the appearance of interferon (a naturally occurring antiviral substance) in the blood (Reyes & Lerner). These data suggest that host resistance to viral infection is severely compromised by forced exercise in a mouse model. Whether these data are applicable to humans is not known.

The effects of exercise on resistance to viral infection depend on when exercise is introduced in relation to the infection (Ilback et al., 1984). In mice, for example, exhaustive swimming training for 6 weeks prior to influenza infection increased survival by 25% compared to nonexercised, infected control animals. In contrast, exhaustive swimming at the time of and for 6 days after infection decreased survival by 33%. Prior exercise training also partially protected against myocardial protein degradation, whereas exercise at the time of infection did not. These data suggest that prior exercise training may protect against viral infection, whereas exercise during the early stages of infection may reduce resistance. It should be noted that in this study the exercised mice ceased training 1 day prior to infection and were permitted to rest during infection. It is not clear whether the protective effect of prior training is maintained when training is continued through the infection.

Effects of exercise on the immune response to bacterial infections have received less attention. From the limited data available, it appears that exercise during bacterial infection is not as detrimental as exercise during viral infection. Survival may be unchanged (Ilback et al., 1984) or enhanced (Cannon & Kluger, 1984) by exercise training before bacterial infection (Figure 1.2). However, few studies compare the immune response to viral and bacterial infections following exercise (Ilback et al., 1984).

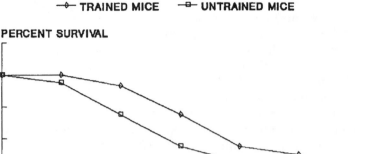

Figure 1.2 Percentage survival in mice infected with *Salmonella typhimurium.* Trained mice were exercise-trained by voluntary running for 16 days prior to infection with *Salmonella typhimurium.* Untrained mice were injected at the same time, without prior exercise training. *p = 0.037 7 days after infection.

Note. From J.G. Cannon and M.J. Kluger, "Exercise Enhances Survival Rate in Mice Infected With *Salmonella Typhimurium,*" *Proceedings of the Society for Experimental Biology and Medicine,* **175**, 518-521, 1984, copyright 1984 by The Society for Experimental Biology and Medicine. Adapted by permission.

Mechanisms Altering Resistance to Infectious Illness

The mechanisms by which intense exercise may alter resistance to infectious illness are not known, and they have received relatively little attention. The immune response to viral and bacterial infections includes antibodies to viral and bacterial proteins, killing activity by certain immune cells, and direct action on foreign agents by soluble factors such as interferon.

In viral infections, a delayed interferon response may permit viral replication, as would a decrease in specific antibodies (Reyes & Lerner, 1976). Other mechanisms that have been suggested include altered T cell function, enhanced spread of virus by the killing of virally infected cells, or increased uptake of virus into cells (Ilback et al., 1989). For example, a 3-fold increase in the number of cytotoxic/suppressor T cells localizing to the heart has been observed in mice exercised 48 hr after infection with coxsackievirus, and this change was correlated with myocardial structural damage (Ilback et al., 1989). An increase in the number of these T cells may suppress normal immune responsiveness.

There is some evidence that soluble serum factors may be involved in exercise-induced immunosuppression during viral infection. For example, in vitro replication of bovine rhinotracheitis virus increased when serum from exercised steers was added to the incubation system (Blecha & Minocha, 1983). Serum cortisol levels increased after exercise in these animals, and addition of hydrocortisone to the assay system (without serum from exercised animals) partially mimicked immunosuppression observed with exercise. It is well known that corticosteroids suppress a variety of immune parameters. It is possible that exercise-induced changes in host defense against infectious illness may involve a combination of factors.

Does Acute Illness Affect Exercise Performance?

Most research on exercise and immunity focuses on the effects of exercise on the body's capacity to mount an immune response. The converse question, whether acute infection and illness influence exercise capacity, has been relatively unexplored. However, there are several reasons and some data (Daniels et al., 1985; Friman, 1977; Roberts, 1986) to suggest that exercise performance may indeed be impaired during infection or illness.

In athletes, decrements in performance have been associated with subclinical viral infection and prolonged recovery after viral infection (Roberts, 1985, 1986). Aerobic exercise capacity during prolonged submaximal work appears to be compromised during febrile viral illness (Daniels et al., 1985), and isometric and isokinetic strength also appear to be adversely affected by viral illness (Daniels et al; Friman, 1977). But the effects of illness are transitory; normal strength and exercise capacity are restored upon recovery from illness (Daniels et al.; Friman).

Certain infections cause disturbances in cellular structure or energy metabolism in a variety of tissues, notably myocardial and skeletal muscle (Cabinian et al., 1990; Woodruff, 1980). Protein degradation and impaired protein synthesis or energy metabolism may limit both exercise capacity and long-term adaptations to exercise training.

Infection causes release of factors that may impair or interfere with normal physiological responses to exercise. For example, the cytokine interleukin 1 (IL-1) is released early in the immune response. IL-1 is pyrogenic (raises core temperature), which may tax thermoregulatory mechanisms and limit the capacity for sustained exercise. IL-1 also increases muscle protein degradation (Hamblin, 1988), possibly limiting muscle adaptations to exercise (see chapter 6).

Practical Considerations

It has been suggested that certain illnesses, including infectious mononucleosis, require extended recovery (up to 6 months) before an athlete resumes intense exercise (Roberts, 1986). Other viral illnesses, such as the common cold without systemic involvement, may not require cessation of training (Roberts, 1986; Simon, 1987). However, impaired strength and exercise capacity during viral infection may lead to musculoskeletal injury in athletes who continue to train during illness (Simon, 1987). Moreover, systemic viral infections may cause structural and functional changes in cardiac and skeletal muscle. Intense exercise during infection may exacerbate illness, leading to complications and, possibly but rarely, death. Roberts (1986) suggested that viral illness with systemic involvement (e.g., fatigue, muscle aches, enlarged lymph nodes) requires 1 month for complete recovery before resumption of intense training. As a general rule, athletes should not train intensely during any infection until the illness is diagnosed by a physician, who can recommend the proper course of treatment and training.

Summary and Conclusions

Competitive endurance athletes appear to suffer elevated rates of infectious illness, especially upper respiratory illness, as a result of intense training or competition. In contrast, "recreational" athletes do not appear to increase their risk of infectious illness through more moderate exercise, such as jogging. The physiological and psychological stress of training and competing at the elite level probably have a combined effect on susceptibility to illness.

Experimental animal models suggest that moderate exercise training prior to experimentally induced viral or bacterial infection enhances resistance, whereas intense exercise at the time of infection reduces resistance. Acute infectious illness in athletes may adversely affect exercise performance, and intense exercise during systemic infection may exacerbate illness. Athletes should not train intensely during acute systemic infection until a medical diagnosis is obtained.

Chapter 2

Overview of the Immune System

The immune system probably developed as a means of self-identification and of maintaining homeostasis. As such, it is exsitely complex, capable of recognizing and defending the body against, theoretically, infinite environmental challenges. The immune system covers the body's responses to foreign or novel molecules, usually proteins, called immunogens; microorganisms, including viruses, bacteria, fungi, and parasites; tumor growth; tissue transplantation; and allergens. The immune response to any challenge requires complex communication and coordination among tissues, cells, and messenger molecules throughout the body.

The literature on exercise and immunology focuses on diverse aspects of immune function (described separately in subsequent chapters). Because of the complexity of the immune system and its nomenclature, I focus here on only those aspects of immune function addressed in the exercise literature.

General Scheme of the Immune Response

A simplified scheme of the immune response to an infectious agent is presented in Figure 2.1. The immune response begins when an invading foreign agent, usually a microorganism, meets and is engulfed by phagocytes, which kill the microbe and degrade its proteins. The foreign proteins are processed by the phagocyte, appearing on the cell surface in combination with the phagocyte's own cell surface proteins. Specialized immune cells, called helper T lymphocytes (T_H), recognize and are activated by the foreign protein on the phagocyte's surface. Upon activation these helper T cells then stimulate other immune cells to proliferate and secrete substances that combat the microorganism. Cytotoxic cells are stimulated to kill the microorganism. Antibodies are produced against the foreign proteins by B lymphocytes, another type of immune cell; antibodies

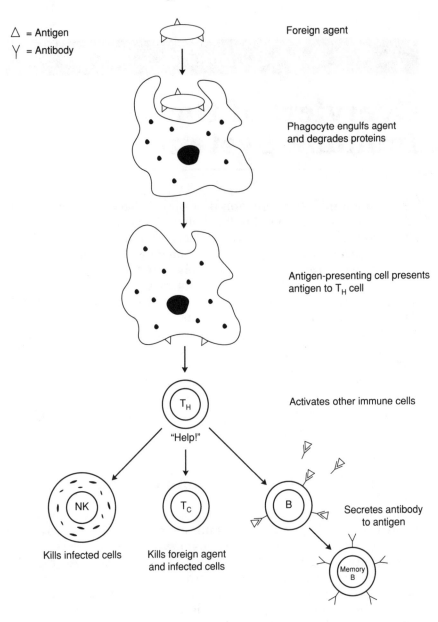

△ = Antigen
Y = Antibody

Foreign agent

Phagocyte engulfs agent
and degrades proteins

Antigen-presenting cell presents
antigen to T$_H$ cell

T$_H$ Activates other immune cells

"Help!"

NK   T$_C$ B   Secretes antibody
                                                 to antigen

Kills infected cells   Kills foreign agent
                                 and infected cells

Memory
B

Figure 2.1   General scheme of the immune response.

neutralize some microbes and stimulate killing by other cells. During the initial encounter with a microbe, "memory" immune cells are generated to respond quickly to subsequent infection by the same microbe, conferring immunity in some instances. The combination of these processes is sufficient to eliminate most microbes; however, in some situations the host's defenses are ineffective or inappropriate.

Innate and Acquired Immunity

The immune response can be divided into two broad functions: innate (natural) immunity and adaptive (acquired) immunity (Table 2.1). Innate immunity is the first aspect of the immune system encountered by an invading microorganism; cells involved in innate immunity can recognize and deal with "nonself" without prior exposure. Innate immunity does not improve with repeated exposure. Adaptive immunity is characterized by specificity to the infectious agent, and it generates "memory" of prior exposure. The adaptive response improves with repeated exposure and is the basis for immunization to prevent disease.

Innate immunity involves three general mechanisms to prevent infection:

Table 2.1   Innate and Acquired Immunity

Innate immunity	Acquired immunity
Physical barriers	Humoral
Skin, epithelial cell barrier	Antibodies
Mucus	Memory
Chemical barriers	Cell-mediated
Complement	T cells
Lysozyme	
pH of bodily fluids	
Acute phase proteins	
Other secretions	
Cells	
Monocytes/macrophages	
Granulocytes	
Natural killer cells	

1. Structural barriers preventing entry of pathogenic organisms
2. Chemical means (pH and soluble factors) that create an inhospitable environment for microorganisms
3. Phagocytic cells that recognize and kill microorganisms

Acquired immunity involves action of immune cells, such as lymphocytes and macrophages, that inactivate and destroy microorganisms by several mechanisms. "Memory" B cells are generated by the first exposure to the foreign agent, and subsequent exposure produces a faster and more effective response.

The acquired immune response can be broadly divided into responses mediated either by humoral agents such as antibodies or by immune cells (cell-mediated immunity, or CMI) that activate other immune cells to combat foreign agents and can directly kill foreign or infected cells.

Cells of the Immune System

Immune cells are found in several lymphoid organs throughout the body and in the blood and lymph circulation. Immature cells proliferate and develop in the bone marrow and then undergo further maturation (differentiation) in primary lymphoid tissues, such as the thymus (T cells) and bone marrow (B cells). Immune cells interact with other cells and foreign proteins in secondary lymphoid tissue in the lymph nodes, spleen, and gut. In lymph nodes throughout the body, foreign proteins (antigens) filtered from lymph are taken up by antigen-presenting cells and presented to lymphocytes to initiate the immune response.

Immune cells migrate between different lymphoid tissues via the circulation and the lymphatic system. Lymphocytes exit the circulation into various lymphoid tissues via specialized venules. It has been estimated that 1% to 2% of the body's total lymphocytes recirculate through the blood every hour (Roitt, Brostoff, & Male, 1989), providing for frequent interaction between foreign proteins and immune cells.

Types of Immune Cells

All cells involved in the immune response arise from a common ancestor, the hemopoietic stem cell found in bone marrow. Three basic lines of immune cells (leukocytes) descend from the stem cell (see Table 2.2): (a) cells of myeloid lineage (monocytes/macrophages and granulocytes); (b) cells of lymphoid lineage (T and B lymphocytes); and (c) "third-population" cells (natural killer, or NK, cells)

(Roitt et al., 1989), although there is uncertainty about the lineage of this third class.

Immune cells display unique cell surface proteins that researchers use to identify, classify, and study these cells, primarily by using

Table 2.2   Circulating Leukocytes and Lymphocytes

Cell	% of circulating leukocytes	Primary function(s)
Granulocyte	60-70	
Neutrophil	>90 of granulocytes	Phagocytosis
Eosinophil	2-5 of granulocytes	Phagocytosis of parasites
Basophil	0.2 of granulocytes	Chemotactic factor production
		Allergic responses
Monocyte	10-15	Phagocytosis
		Antigen presentation
		Cytokine production
		Cytotoxicity
Lymphocyte	20-25	Lymphocyte activation
		Lymphokine production
		Antigen recognition
		Antibody production
		Memory
		Cytotoxicity

Cell	% of lymphocytes	Function(s)
T cell	60-75	Lymphocyte regulation
T_H (CD4)	60-70 of T cells	Lymphokine secretion
		Antigen recognition
		B cell proliferation
T_C/T_S (CD8)	30-40 of T cells	Cytotoxicity
		Lymphocyte suppression
B cell	5-15	Antibody production
		Memory
LGL/NK	10-20	Cytotoxicity
		Lymphokine production

Note. Data from Roitt, Brostoff, and Male (1989, pp. 2.2-2.18).

monoclonal antibodies to the proteins. Many of these cell surface proteins have specific functions, such as receptors. By recent international agreement, these proteins (and the cells they identify) are now designated by the prefix CD (cluster designation) (Roitt et al., 1989).

Myeloid Immune Cells

Monocytes and macrophages are phagocytic and antigen-presenting myeloid cells derived from a promonocyte precursor in bone marrow. Monocytes are found in the circulation but can localize to tissues during injury, inflammation, and infection. Once in tissues, these cells differentiate further and are termed macrophages.

The monocyte is a relatively large (10 to 18 μm) cell that is involved in the early stages of the innate immune response, primarily via phagocytosis (ingestion) of microorganisms and presentation of antigen to lymphocytes. The monocyte/macrophage kills ingested microorganisms by releasing proteases from lysosomes and by generating molecules such as hydrogen peroxide and oxygen radicals that are toxic to microorganisms. Once activated, the monocyte/macrophage also produces several soluble factors that activate lymphocytes. Monocytes/macrophages may also kill tumor and virally infected cells.

Polymorphonuclear granulocytes (polymorphs) are large (10 to 20 μm) granule-containing leukocytes, which are among the first cells to encounter foreign organisms. There are three types of polymorphs: neutrophils, which comprise the majority of circulating leukocytes; eosinophils; and basophils. Each can be characterized by a distinct morphology and staining with certain histochemical dyes.

Neutrophils, the most prevalent of the leukocytes, are phagocytic cells that kill ingested microorganisms by releasing proteases from cytoplasmic granules and by generating toxic molecules such as hydrogen peroxide and oxygen radicals. Neutrophils are attracted to the sites of infection by chemotactic factors produced by other leukocytes; they can adhere to and move through capillary walls to reach the site of infection or inflammation.

Eosinophils comprise a small percentage of circulating leukocytes and are capable of phagocytosis of microorganisms. Eosinophils are most active in resistance to parasitic infections, and they play a minor role in asthma. Basophils and mast cells comprise a very small percentage of circulating leukocytes and are primarily involved in allergic and inflammatory reactions.

Lymphoid Immune Cells

T lymphocytes, or T cells, are small (6 to 10 μm) lymphoid cells distinguished by the T cell receptor (TCR, CD3) displayed on the cell surface. T cells are intimately involved in initiating and regulating most immune responses because of their ability to modulate the activity of several immune cells. Examples of this modulation include the activation of B cells to proliferate and produce antibody; the killing of tumor and virally infected cells; and secretion of soluble factors that modulate the activity of other immune cells.

T_H *and* T_C *Cells.*   There are two distinct subpopulations of T lymphocytes, the helper/inducer T (T_H) cell and the cytotoxic/suppressor T (T_C/T_S) cell. These cells can be distinguished by function and by cell surface proteins, notably CD4 on T_H cells and CD8 on T_C/T_S cells.

T_H (CD4) cells regulate much of the immune response, especially of B and other T cells. T_H cells secrete soluble factors that stimulate B and T cell proliferation and differentiation. Activation of T_H cells is an essential first step for most immune responses. Factors secreted by T_H cells also stimulate the killing activity of other immune cells (see later discussion).

T_C/T_S (CD8) cells are regulatory and cytotoxic cells, which can be further subdivided by function and other cell surface proteins. T_C cells can kill a variety of targets, including some tumor cells, virally infected cells, and parasites. T_S cells are involved in regulating B and other T cells by suppressing certain functions; this may be important in turning off the immune response once completed. The overall interaction and coordination of the different types of T cells provide for fine control over the immune response.

B Cells.   B cells produce antibodies that appear on the B cell surface as receptors for antigen (foreign proteins); soluble antibody is also found in serum or other body fluids. B cells are identified by the markers CD19, CD20, and CD22 (Roitt et al., 1989).

Under normal conditions, resting B cells are small (6 to 10 μm). Upon activation by T cells, B cells proliferate and differentiate into plasma cells producing large amounts of antibody. B cells carry "memory" of earlier encounters with antigen. Subsequent exposure results in a faster and greater production of antibody directed against the antigen. Each B or plasma cell produces antibody that recognizes only a single antigen.

Third-Population Immune Cells

The exact lineage of third-population cells is uncertain, but it is generally accepted that they arise from the common bone marrow stem cell (Roitt et al., 1989). These cells include the large granular lymphocytes (LGL), which exhibit NK activity. LGL are identified histologically as large lymphocytes (15 μm) with many cytoplasmic granules and by cell surface markers such as CD16 and CD56. LGL can recognize, bind to, and kill some tumor and virally infected cells. LGL also exhibit antibody-dependent, cell-mediated cytotoxicity (ADCC).

Antigen-presenting cells (APC) are a heterogeneous population of cell types able to process and present antigen to immune cells, an important step in initiating the immune response. Phagocytic cells such as monocytes/macrophages and dendritic cells, as well as some B cells and some nonimmune cells, can present antigen. APC appear in the circulation and in a variety of lymphoid tissues, including skin, lymph nodes, spleen, and thymus (Roitt et al., 1989).

Antibodies and Immunoglobulins

Immunoglobulins (Ig) are glycoproteins produced and secreted by B and plasma cells. Ig are found in serum and other body fluids. An antibody is an Ig molecule that reacts with a specific antigen; all antibodies are Ig, but not all Ig exhibit antibody activity. Antibodies are important to antigen recognition and memory of earlier exposure to specific antigens. Antibodies on the B cell surface act as receptors for antigen, which is important in initiating the acquired immune response.

Antibodies serve many functions:

- Neutralizing bacterial toxins and some viruses
- Immobilizing and agglutinizing (clumping) microbes
- Facilitating binding of antigen to phagocytes
- Stimulating complement killing of microbes
- Stimulating ADCC

Ig Structure and Recognition of Antigen

The basic Ig molecule consists of four polypeptide chains, two light and two heavy chains, linked together by disulfide bonds (Figure 2.2). The two ends of the molecule have different functions: The Fab end has a specific three-dimensional structure for binding to antigen, whereas the Fc end binds to receptors on immune cells. This bifunctional structure is important to immune cell recognition of foreign antigen.

Each B or plasma cell produces a single type of antibody to a particular antigen. Upon exposure to a specific antigen, a particular

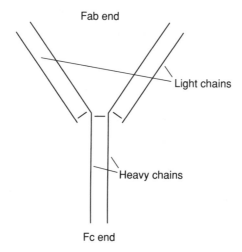

Figure 2.2   Basic structure of an immunoglobulin molecule.

B cell proliferates and differentiates into myriad mature plasma cells secreting antibody against the antigen. Because each pathogenic organism may express several different antigens and several antibodies may be directed against each antigen, production of antibody is usually a highly effective immune response.

There are five classes of Ig in higher mammals, which are similar in basic structure and function but differ in size, composition, and specific functions. The five classes are referred to by letter: IgA, IgD, IgG, IgE, and IgM. The relative amounts and distributions of Ig classes also differ; for example, IgG is predominant in serum and IgA is most prevalent in mucosal fluids.

Phagocytosis

Phagocytosis is an important early step in the immune response. As mentioned, many cells are capable of phagocytosis, including monocytes/macrophages, neutrophils, and various APC located in tissues. Phagocytosis involves five basic steps:

1. Localization to the site of infection
2. Binding to the organism
3. Ingestion of the organism
4. Killing
5. Degradation of the organism

After degradation the foreign antigens are processed and displayed on the phagocyte's cell surface. Presentation of antigen to T cells is essential to the next phase of the immune response, T cell activation.

Soluble Factors in the Immune Response

The immune response involves many soluble factors, which act in several ways:

- To activate immune cells
- As chemical messengers between different immune cells
- As agents able to neutralize or kill foreign agents
- To regulate the immune response

Cytokines

Cytokines are polypeptides that are involved in communication between lymphoid cells (Cohen, 1990; Hamblin, 1988). Lymphokines are cytokines released by lymphoid cells (T and B cells, large granular lymphocytes), and monokines are molecules of similar function released by monocytes/macrophages. Cytokines may also be released by other cells, such as fibroblasts. Cytokines are soluble factors that act primarily to stimulate immune cell growth and differentiation and to activate immune cell function. These molecules may act alone or with other molecules, sometimes synergistically. Cytokines are involved in virtually all aspects of immune function, and they may also act on cells outside the immune system, such as cells of the neuroendocrine system. In addition to cytokines, there are myriad recently identified growth-stimulating and inhibiting factors that interact with cytokines to influence immune function.

There are several general classes of cytokines, each with diverse functions (Table 2.3). Molecules in the same class are not necessarily related in structure or function. Some cytokines exist in isoforms, which may or may not have different functions. The general classes of cytokines that have been characterized are interleukins (IL), interferons (IFN), tumor necrosis factors (TNF), and colony-stimulating factors (CSF).

Interleukins

Interleukins are lymphoid cell growth factors secreted primarily by T cells but also by monocytes/macrophages, B cells, and LGL. At present, at least 12 types of IL have been identified in the human;

Table 2.3   Cytokines

Cytokine	Primary producer(s)	Immune actions
IL-1	Activated monocytes, macrophages and APC	Increase IL-2r expression T_H activation Increase B cell proliferation Increase TNF, IL-6, CSF
IL-2	Activated T_H cells NK cells	T cell activation Increase IL-2r expression Increase IFN Stimulate B cell proliferation Monocyte activation Stimulate NK cytotoxicity
IL-3	Activated T_H cells	Granulocyte and monocyte differentiation
IL-4	Activated T_H cells	Stimulate T cell growth and B cell differentiation
IL-5	Activated T_H cells	Stimulate plasma cell growth
IL-6	Activated T_H cells and fibroblasts	Stimulate Ig secretion
IFNα and IFNβ	Virally infected cells	Stimulate macrophage and NK killing Stimulate antigen presentation
IFNγ	Activated T_H cells and NK cells	Stimulate monocyte and NK killing Inhibit viral replication
TNFα	Monocytes and T, B, and NK cells	Enhanced tumor cell killing Antiviral activity
TNFβ	T cells	Enhanced tumor cell killing
GM-CSF	Activated T cells	Stimulate granulocyte and eosinophil differentiation
G-CSF	Activated monocytes	Granulocyte differentiation
M-CSF	Fibroblasts	Stimulate macrophage differentiation

Note. Data from Cohen (1990); Hamblin (1988); and Roitt, Brostoff, and Male (1989).

IL-1 through IL-6 have been most completely characterized. These molecules are not necessarily related in structure or function.

IL-1 is produced by monocytes/macrophages and exerts a wide range of actions, such as stimulation of various processes:

- IL-2 production and IL-2 receptor expression on T_H cells
- Monocyte/macrophage production of other cytokines, such as TNF and IL-6
- B cell proliferation and differentiation
- Neutrophil activation
- Killing by NK cells

IL-1 is also involved in inflammation, stimulation of prostaglandin secretion, elevation of body temperature, proteolysis of muscle proteins, and leukocyte infiltration at tissue sites of injury or infection.

IL-2 is produced by T_H and NK cells. IL-2 stimulates many immune parameters, such as:

- Proliferation of T and B cells
- Expression of the IL-2 receptor on T and B cells
- Release of other cytokines, such as IFN
- Proliferation and killing by NK cells

Expression of the IL-2 receptor is an essential early step in the initiation of the immune response. IL-2 receptors are found in low concentration on resting immune cells; upon activation by IL-1, T_H cells express more IL-2 receptors and secrete more IL-2, which in turn increases the number of IL-2 receptors on B cells, NK cells, and monocytes/macrophages.

IL-3 is a hematopoietic growth factor produced by activated T_H cells. IL-3 stimulates differentiation of myeloid cells (granulocytes and monocytes). IL-4, IL-5, and IL-6 are produced mainly by T_H cells and act as B cell growth factors, although IL-4 also stimulates T cell growth, IL-5 is involved in eosinophil differentiation, and IL-6 is involved in inflammation (Le & Vilcek, 1989; Roitt et al., 1989).

Interferons

The three distinct types of interferons (α, β, and γ) are unrelated in structure and function. IFNα and IFNβ are released from virally infected cells, and they exert antiviral activity by stimulating NK and macrophage killing of infected cells, enhancing antigen presentation of viral proteins, and possibly inhibiting viral replication (Roitt et al., 1989). IFNγ is produced by activated T_H and

NK cells and exerts weak antiviral activity. IFNγ activates many immune cells, including monocytes/macrophages and T_C and B cells.

Tumor Necrosis Factors

Two closely related types of TNF have been identified: TNFα (cachectin) and TNFβ (lymphotoxin). Both exert cytotoxic activity against tumor cells. TNFα is produced by monocytes and T, B, and NK cells. TNFα activates macrophage killing of tumor cells and also has antiviral activity. There are also harmful effects from high levels of TNFα, including inflammation and cachexia (muscle wasting in cancer or prolonged infections). TNFβ is produced by activated T cells and exerts both cytostatic (growth-inhibiting) and cytotoxic (killing) activity against tumor cells.

Colony-Stimulating Factors

The three main classes of CSF all stimulate division and differentiation of myeloid cells from the hemopoietic stem cell. Granulocyte-macrophage CSF (GM-CSF) is produced by activated T cells and stimulates differentiation of granulocytes, macrophages, and eosinophils. Granulocyte CSF (G-CSF) is secreted by activated monocytes and macrophages and stimulates granulocyte differentiation. Macrophage CSF (M-CSF) is produced by monocytes and fibroblasts and stimulates macrophage differentiation.

Other Soluble Factors

Body fluids contain soluble factors, such as complement and acute phase proteins (APP), that act early in the immune response to counteract invading microorganisms.

Complement

Complement, a complex system of at least 20 proteins found in serum, was one of the first soluble factors identified as important in the immune response. The complement system is a central feature in resistance to bacteria and in the inflammatory process; complement may also act in resistance to viral and parasitic infections. Complement acts primarily to stimulate phagocytosis and antigen presentation, as well as being involved in the killing of infected cells.

Acute Phase Proteins

APP, or acute phase reactants (APR), are several unrelated serum proteins synthesized in the liver that are part of the innate immune response. Concentrations of APP may increase up to 100 times following infection or inflammation. C-reactive protein (CRP) is the predominant APP.

APP act in several ways during inflammation and infection. They are chemotactic for leukocytes, enhancing their migration to sites of infection or injury. CRP binds to some bacterial proteins, activating complement and phagocytosis. Other APP, the proteinase inhibitors, limit proteolysis of muscle and other tissue proteins, whereas metal-binding proteins bind iron and copper-containing compounds, which may inhibit bacterial growth by reducing availability of these metals. APP levels may be increased during inflammation (e.g., tissue damage) in the absence of infection.

Immune Response to Tumor Cells

The immune system plays a dual role in the body's defense against cancer—first, by "immunosurveillance" against spontaneously arising tumor cells and, second, by killing or checking (or both) the growth of tumor cells after they appear. Initiation of the immune response to tumor cells is in many ways similar to the early cell-mediated response to infectious agents and involves interaction of several cytokines (Table 2.3). APC present tumor cell antigens to T and B cells. Activated T_H cells secrete cytokines, which stimulate cytotoxic activity of T_C and NK cells as well as macrophages. Cytokines also stimulate B cell production of antibody directed against the tumor antigens. Cytokines may also exhibit direct cytostatic and cytotoxic activities on tumor cells.

Cytotoxic activity is exhibited by T_C cells, NK cells, macrophages, and neutrophils. The general mechanisms of killing by T_C and NK cells appear to be similar, although there are differences in the cytotoxic molecules involved. Binding of the cytotoxic (effector) cell to the tumor (target) cell is a requisite first step. Once bound, the cytotoxic cell inserts "pores," or ringlike structures, into the tumor cell membrane and injects cytotoxic molecules, which ultimately rupture the target cell membrane.

Summary and Conclusions

The immune system is extremely complex, capable of distinguishing "self" from "nonself" and of generating "memory" of prior exposure to foreign agents. The immune response to a challenge involves coordination of many cell types, soluble factors, and messenger molecules located throughout the body. Three basic types of cells (leukocytes) are involved in the immune response: monocytes/macrophages and granulocytes; lymphocytes; and "third-population" cells such as natural killer and antigen-presenting cells. Other major mechanisms of host resistance include soluble factors secreted by various cells, such as antibody specific to a foreign antigen; cytokines, which activate and regulate various immune cells; and acute phase proteins, which enhance activity of immune cells. Certain immune cells (cytotoxic T lymphocytes, monocytes/macrophages, natural killer cells) are also capable of recognizing and killing tumor cells, providing "immunosurveillance" against spontaneous neoplastic growth.

Chapter 3

Exercise and Leukocytes: Number, Distribution, and Proliferation

Exercise causes profound changes in the number and distribution of circulating leukocytes and may also induce changes in lymphocyte proliferation. Redistribution of leukocytes has been attributed to hormonal changes occurring during and immediately after exercise. Exercise-induced changes in leukocyte number, distribution, and proliferation are largely transitory, and it is unclear whether immune function is influenced by these changes.

Leukocyte Number and Cell Distribution

Leukocytosis (increase in circulating leukocyte number) is one of the most striking and consistent changes observed during exercise (for review, see McCarthy & Dale, 1988). Circulating leukocyte number may increase up to 4 times, may continue to rise after cessation of exercise, and may remain elevated for prolonged periods (up to 24 hr) after some types of exercise. In general, the magnitude of leukocytosis appears to be directly related to exercise intensity and duration and inversely related to fitness level; exercise duration may be the most important factor (McCarthy & Dale). The increase in leukocyte number is due predominantly to increases in neutrophil and, to a lesser extent, lymphocyte counts, although monocyte numbers also increase.

Resting Leukocyte Number in Athletes

It has been suggested that well-trained athletes exhibit low resting leukocyte numbers (Davidson, Robertson, Galea, & Maughan, 1987; Green, Kaplan, Rabin, Stanitski, & Zdziarski, 1981). For example, Green et al. reported that 4 of 20 runners had low leukocyte numbers (below 4.3×10^3 per µl; normal range is 4 to 11×10^3 per µl). Similarly, leukocyte counts of less than 5×10^3 per μl were reported in 5 of 9 long-distance runners (Moorthy & Zimmerman, 1978).

However, most studies comparing trained athletes with nonathletes and comparing the same individuals before and after training report no significant effect of training on resting leukocyte numbers (Busse, Anderson, Hanson, & Folts, 1980; Ferry, Picard, Duvallet, Weill, & Rieu, 1990; Gimenez et al., 1987; Lewicki, Tchorzewski, Denys, Kowalska, & Golinska, 1987; Nehlsen-Cannarella et al., 1991; Oshida, Yamanouchi, Hayamizu, & Sato, 1988; Priest, Oei, & Moorehead, 1982; Soppi, Varjo, Eskola, & Laitinen, 1982). Virtually all papers report clinically normal values (see McCarthy & Dale, 1988).

Exercise-Induced Changes in Leukocyte Number

A large body of literature shows increases in leukocyte number following a variety of exercises, ranging in duration from a few seconds (100-yd run) to hours (marathon running, marching). The magnitude of increases varies and is determined by a combination of exercise intensity and duration. For example, counts increase up to 2 times after exercise lasting less than 1 hr, 2 to 3 times after exercise of 1 to 2 hr, and up to 4 times after more than 2 hr of exercise (McCarthy & Dale, 1988).

Exercise Leukocytosis in Athletes

Leukocytosis has been observed during exercise in trained humans and other species, such as horses and dogs. Leukocyte number may remain elevated for several hours after prolonged exercise (Davidson et al., 1987; Nieman, Berk, et al., 1989). For example, in runners leukocyte number increased from a resting level of 5.4 to 13.7×10^3 per μl immediately after a 3-hr treadmill run at marathon race pace, and further to 15×10^3 per μl 1.5 hr after. Leukoycte counts remained elevated (11.8×10^3 per μl) 6 hr postexercise but returned to preexercise levels by 21 hr after the run (Figure 3.1) (Nieman, Berk et al.).

In contrast, during very long exercise, such as a 24-hr march, leukocyte number increased progressively up to 16 hr, then decreased and remained slightly below resting levels for 62 hr after the march (Galun et al., 1987). Decreased leukocyte count after very prolonged exercise may be due to catecholamine depletion (see later discussion).

Shorter exercise also increases leukocyte number in trained athletes. With exercise lasting less than 1 hr, leukocyte number

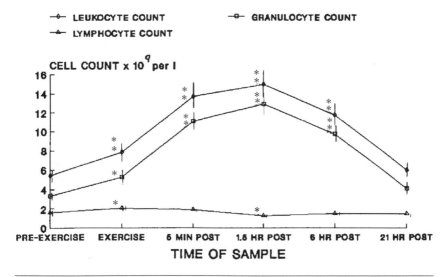

Figure 3.1 Leukocyte number before and after a 3-hr run. Marathon runners ran on a treadmill for 3 hr at race pace. Blood was collected before and up to 21 hr after the run, and leukocyte subsets were determined by flow cytometry. Bars represent standard errors of the mean (SEM). $*p < .05$; $**p < .01$ compared to preexercise values.

Note. From "Effects of Long-Endurance Running on Immune System Parameters and Lymphocyte Function in Experienced Marathoners" by D.C. Nieman, L.S. Berk, M. Simpson-Westerberg, K. Arabatzis, S. Youngberg, S.A. Tan, J.W. Lee, and W.C. Eby, 1989, International Journal of Sports Medicine, **10**, p. 320. Copyright 1989 by Georg Thieme Verlag. Adapted by permission.

rises progressively with exercise intensity (Gimenez, Mohan-Kumar, Humbert, de Talance, & Buisine, 1986). Compared to endurance exercise, brief exercise causes less of an increase in leukocyte number and faster restoration of resting leukocyte count after exercise. Trained male and female runners exhibit similar leukocyte, neutrophil, and lymphocyte responses to endurance exercise (Davidson et al., 1987; Wells, Stern, & Hecht, 1982).

Exercise Leukocytosis in Nonathletes

Untrained subjects also exhibit leukocytosis during and after various types of exercise. The magnitude of exercise-induced leukocytosis in untrained subjects is similar to that in athletes when exercise is at the same relative work rate (i.e., the same percentage of $\dot{V}O_2$max; Oshida et al., 1988). However, athletes exhibit less of an increase in leukocyte number at the same absolute work rate, which is generally lower relative to maximum capacity (Gimenez et al., 1987). Short-term exercise training in previously untrained individuals does not alter the magnitude of leukocytosis during maximal exercise (Busse et al., 1980; Soppi et al., 1982).

Granulocyte Number

Granulocyte number increases markedly after strenuous or prolonged exercise but may not change after brief or low-intensity exercise. The increase is greatest after intense prolonged exercise. For example, granulocyte number was unchanged after uphill walking at 50% of VO_2max (Smith et al., 1989), increased by 26% after 10 min of (presumably maximal) stair climbing in adolescent track athletes (Christensen & Hill, 1987), and increased more than 300% after a marathon (Figure 3.1) (Moorthy & Zimmerman, 1978; Nieman, Berk, et al., 1989). Granulocyte number may remain elevated for several hours after intense prolonged exercise (Nieman, Berk, et al.).

Leukocyte Trafficking During Exercise

Under resting conditions, less than half of the body's mature leukocytes are circulating in the vascular system. The remainder are sequestered in underperfused microvasculature in the lungs, liver, and spleen. The exact mechanisms by which leukocytes are released into the circulation during exercise are unknown, but most likely they involve mechanical factors such as increased cardiac output and perfusion of the microvasculature as well as changes in the interactions between leukocytes and endothelial cells of the capillaries (Foster, Martyn, Rangno, Hogg, & Pardy, 1986; McCarthy & Dale, 1988; Muir et al., 1984). Immature leukocytes may also be released from the bone marrow. Many of these changes are under hormonal control (see later discussion).

It has been suggested that some of the leukocytes mobilized during exercise localize to damaged muscle fibers afterward (Smith et al., 1989). This is consistent with the observation that leukocyte number is higher after exercise with a large eccentric component compared to exercise with relatively little eccentric activity. (Eccentric exercise requires the muscle to lengthen while generating force and is associated with muscle fiber damage and delayed muscle soreness.)

It is unlikely that most of the leukocytes mobilized during exercise localize to muscle tissue after exercise, for the following reasons.

First, neutrophils are the major leukocytes recruited into the circulation during eccentric exercise (Smith et al., 1989), whereas histological evidence shows monocytes and T_H cells to be the major cells localizing to damaged skeletal muscle fibers after eccentric exercise (Round, Jones, & Cambridge, 1987). Second, significant leukocytosis occurs during and after concentric exercise, which does not cause muscle damage. It is possible that some of the leukocytes, particularly monocytes and T_H cells recruited during exercise, localize to damaged muscle fibers, but this cannot fully explain the eventual return of leukocyte number toward resting levels after exercise.

Lymphocyte Number and Subset Distribution

Resting lymphocyte number is usually normal in athletes (McCarthy & Dale, 1988; Oshida et al., 1988), although low lymphocyte counts have been reported in marathon runners (Green et al., 1981). For example, 10 of 20 marathon runners had resting lymphocyte counts of less than 1.5×10^3 per μl (normal range is 1.5 to 4.0×10^3 per μl). However, it was also noted that at least 5 athletes had completed marathon or other long runs within 3 days of blood sampling. It is possible that the low lymphocyte counts reflected a long-lasting effect of the last run; lymphocyte number has been shown to decrease below resting levels after distance running (see later discussion).

Lymphocytosis (increase in lymphocyte number) occurs during and immediately after exercise under a variety of conditions, from 10 min of stair climbing to marathon running. The magnitude of increase in lymphocyte number is generally less than for granulocyte number (Figure 3.1). Lymphocyte number returns to resting levels early in recovery after exercise, before resting granulocyte number is restored. However, lymphocyte number may decrease below resting level before returning to preexercise values (see later discussion).

As with leukocytes, lymphocyte number rises progressively with increasing work rate, and the magnitude of lymphocytosis is related to exercise intensity. However, in contrast to leukocytosis, duration may not be an important determinant. For example, similar lymphocytosis was observed during maximal cycle tests of different durations (7 and 25 min), and in a longer test (45 min) lymphocyte count plateaued after 15 min (Gimenez et al., 1986).

The degree of lymphocytosis during exercise appears to depend on an interaction of exercise intensity and fitness level. During moderate or very brief (1 min) exercise, lymphocyte number remains unchanged (Rose & Bloomberg, 1989; Smith et al., 1989) or increases up to 50% above resting levels (Oshida et al., 1988). During intense or prolonged exercise, lymphocyte number increases 30% to 100% above resting counts in trained athletes and 70% to 200% in untrained individuals (Gimenez et al., 1987; Hedfors, Holm, & Ohnell, 1976; Hedfors, Holm, Ivansen, & Wahren, 1983; Oshida et al.; Soppi et al., 1982).

Whereas leukocyte and neutrophil numbers gradually return to baseline levels after exercise, lymphocyte numbers may decrease below resting levels before returning to normal after endurance exercise (Nieman, Berk, et al., 1989; Tvede et al., 1989). For example, in marathon runners lymphocyte count was 20% lower 1.5 hr after a 3-hr run compared to preexercise levels. Lymphocyte number returned to normal by 6 hr, although leukocyte and granulocyte numbers remained elevated at this time (Nieman, Berk, et al., 1989). These data suggest that different factors may influence lymphocyte and granulocyte redistribution during and after exercise.

Exercise and Lymphocyte Subsets

The relative proportions of lymphocyte subsets (T, B, and NK cells) obtained at rest do not differ between athletes and nonathletes (Oshida et al., 1988) or after moderate training in previously sedentary individuals (Nehlsen-Cannarella et al., 1991), suggesting that exercise training has no long-term effect on lymphocyte distribution.

Various lymphocyte subsets may respond differently to exercise. In general, all subsets increase in number, but B and NK cells may increase in number proportionately more than T cells. The ratio of T_H to T_S cells may change, because there are disproportionate increases in T cell subsets (Table 3.1; Figure 3.2). Monocyte number also increases during and after exercise. The end result is that the percentages of the subsets relative to each other and to total lymphocytes change.

In addition, there may be individual variation in the lymphocyte subset response to exercise, which may partially explain inconsistencies in the literature. For example, changes in T_H and T_S cell numbers were reported after moderate exercise (60 min at 60% $\dot{V}O_2max$) only on the first of two testing sessions spaced 3 weeks apart (Ricken, Rieder, Hauck, & Kindermann, 1990). These results may have been due to subject unfamiliarity with or anxiety about exercise testing on the first occasion and subsequently a more accurate measure of lymphocyte subsets would have been obtained during exercise in the second session.

Table 3.1   Summary of Exercise and T Cell Subsets

Exercise duration intensity	Effect in athletes	Effect in nonathletes
Brief; low	—	No change
Brief; high	Increase T 20%-200% Increase T_H 15%-70% Increase T_S 15%-200%	Increase T_H 70% Increase T_S 200%
Long; low	No change in T Decrease T_H 15%-25% Increase T_S 25% Decrease T_H: T_S	No change in T or TS Decrease T_H 15%-25% Decrease T_H: T_S
Long; high	No change in T or T_H Decrease T_S 30% Increase T_H: T_S	—

Note. Data represent percent changes in total T cell and subset numbers compared to preexercise values, measured immediately after exercise of varying duration and intensity. Brief = <30 min; long = ≥30 min; low intensity = <75% VO_2max; high intensity = ≥75% VO_2max.

Data from Christensen and Hill (1987); Moorthy and Zimmerman (1978); Nieman, Berk, Simpson-Westerberg, Arabatzis, Youngberg, Tan, Lee, and Eby (1989); Oshida, Yamanouchi, Hayamizu, and Sato (1988); Steel, Evans, and Smith (1974).

T Cells

Brief maximal exercise recruits T cells into the circulation so that absolute T cell number increases up to 150% following exercise (Table 3.1 and Figure 3.2) (Bieger, Weiss, Michel, & Weicker, 1980; Christensen & Hill, 1987; Espersen et al., 1990; Ferry et al., 1990; Lewicki, Tchorzewski, Majewska, Nowak, & Baj, 1988). Normal T cell number is generally restored soon after exercise, although the number may decrease below baseline before returning to pre-exercise level (Espersen et al.). The number increases more in untrained than in trained individuals after brief, maximal exercise (e.g., $\dot{V}O_2$max test) (Ferry et al.). Both T_H and T_S cell numbers increase, but the increase in T_H cell count is smaller. As a result, the T_H:T_S ratio may decrease by 30% to 50%, but it is restored by 2 hr postexercise (Lewicki et al., 1988).

In contrast, T and T_H cell numbers remain unchanged following intense prolonged exercise (e.g., marathon running) (Gmunder et al.,

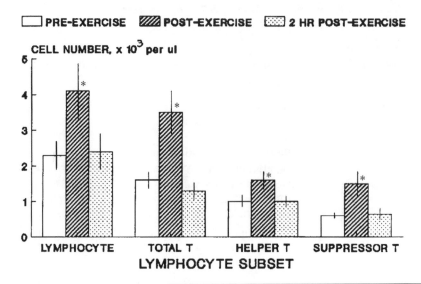

Figure 3.2   Changes in T cell subset numbers after exercise. Trained endurance cyclists performed an incremental cycling test to maximum (average time 19.3 min). Total lymphocyte and T cell subset numbers were determined by indirect immunofluoresence using monoclonal antibodies as specific cell markers. Although the absolute numbers of all cell types increased after exercise, the relative percentages remained fairly constant, except for an increased percentage of T_S cells. The T_H:T_S ratio decreased from 1.5 to 1.0 immediately after exercise but returned to the preexercise level by 2 hr after exercise. Bars represent SEM. *$p <$ .01 compared to preexercise values.

Note. From "Effect of Maximal Physical Exercise on T-Lymphocyte Subpopulations and on Interleukin-1 (IL 1) and Interleukin-2 (IL 2) Production in Vitro" by R. Lewicki, H. Tchorzewski, E. Majewska, Z. Nowak, and Z. Baj, 1988, *International Journal of Sports Medicine*, **9**, p. 115. Copyright 1988 by Georg Thieme Verlag. Adapted by permission.

1988; Moorthy & Zimmerman, 1978; Nieman, Berk, et al., 1989). T_S number may decrease and remain low for up to 21 hr after marathon running; because T_H cell number does not change, the T_H:T_S ratio increases during this time (Nieman, Berk, et al., 1989). Normal values are restored at some point after intense prolonged exercise, because distance runners exhibit normal resting T cell subset distribution (Davidson et al., 1987; Oshida et al., 1988).

B Cells

B cell number increases dramatically during exercise but quickly returns to baseline level afterward (Bieger et al., 1980; Christensen &

Hill, 1987; Espersen et al., 1990; Ferry et al., 1990; Nieman, Berk, et al., 1989; Steel, Evans, & Smith, 1974). Compared to untrained individuals, athletes may exhibit a smaller increase in B cell number during brief maximal exercise (Ferry et al.). B cell number changes only slightly during intense endurance exercise (Nieman, Berk, et al.).

Exercise and NK Cell Number

Exercise causes profound changes in both the percentage and number of circulating NK cells. NK cell percentage relative to total lymphocytes increases 50% to 300% following brief (<30 min) submaximal and maximal as well as prolonged (>45 min) submaximal exercise (Brahmi, Thomas, Park, Park, & Dowdeswell, 1985; Edwards et al., 1984; Espersen et al., 1990; Fiatarone et al., 1988; Kotani et al., 1987; Lewicki et al., 1988; Pedersen et al., 1988, 1990; Tvede et al., 1989). The increase is transitory, with NK percentage returning to resting level by 1 to 2 hr after exercise (Brahmi et al., 1985; Pedersen et al., 1988; Tvede et al.). In contrast, NK percentage does not change immediately after intense endurance exercise (Berk et al., 1990; Mackinnon, Chick, van As, & Tomasi, 1988) but may decrease by 50% during recovery, from 1 to 21 hr after exercise (Berk et al.; Mackinnon et al., 1988).

Changes in NK cell number appear similar to those for NK percentage. NK cell number increases during and immediately after brief submaximal, maximal, and prolonged submaximal exercise (Edwards et al., 1984; Espersen et al., 1990; Kotani et al., 1987; Lewicki et al., 1988; Pedersen et al., 1988, 1990; Tvede et al., 1989). It remains unchanged during or immediately following intense prolonged exercise (Berk et al., 1990; Mackinnon et al., 1988).

Postexercise recovery of NK cell number is complex. NK cell number may decrease 50% (Espersen et al., 1990) or return to normal after brief maximal exercise (Lewicki et al., 1988); may remain elevated after prolonged submaximal exercise (Pedersen et al., 1990); or may decrease by 50% and remain low for up to 21 hr after intense endurance exercise (Berk et al., 1990). NK cell number returns to normal values by 24 hr after all types of exercise (Espersen et al., 1990; Mackinnon et al., 1988). It appears that NK cells are selectively mobilized into the circulation during exercise and then removed after.

Exercise and Monocyte Number

Resting monocyte number is clinically normal in male and female marathon runners (Davidson et al., 1987). Monocyte number may increase markedly during and after intense exercise of both short and long duration; increases of 100% and 50%, respectively, have been noted (Bieger et al., 1980; Christensen & Hill, 1987; Davidson et al.; Espersen et al., 1990; Lewicki et al., 1987; Nieman, Berk, et al., 1989). The magnitude of increase in monocyte number appears to be related to fitness level and exercise duration, although this has not been extensively studied. Because monocytes secrete a number of cytokines, recruitment of monocytes into the circulation may account for increases in these factors during exercise (see chapter 6).

Mechanisms Underlying Changes in Leukocyte Distribution

There is strong evidence to implicate stress hormones as mediators of exercise-induced changes in leukocyte number and subset redistribution. It has long been known that hormones such as epinephrine and cortisol influence leukocyte distribution between the circulation and various body compartments, such as the liver, spleen, and bone marrow. Leukocytosis occurring during exercise has been simulated by exogenous administration of epinephrine at appropriate concentrations seen with exercise (Muir et al., 1984). Leukocytosis during exercise may be abrogated by β-adrenergic blockade during exercise (Ahlborg & Ahlborg, 1970), although other studies have reported inconsistencies (reviewed by McCarthy & Dale, 1988).

Increases in both epinephrine and cortisol are a function of exercise intensity relative to individual exercise capacity, with an apparent threshold of 60% $\dot{V}O_2$max for release of epinephrine (Brooks & Fahey, 1985). There is more individual variability in the glucocorticoid response to exercise. Exercise training results in lower responses of circulating epinephrine and cortisol to the same exercise (Brooks & Fahey). Epinephrine level increases during exercise and returns to baseline levels quickly (within 30 min), whereas cortisol often exhibits a lag before increasing during exercise and may continue to increase or remain elevated longer after cessation of exercise (McCarthy & Dale, 1988).

A high correlation between serum cortisol levels and leukocytosis after exercise has been reported (Eskola et al., 1978; Moorthy & Zimmerman, 1978; Nieman, Berk, et al., 1989). For example, increases in leukocyte and granulocyte numbers were significantly correlated with an increase in serum cortisol concentration (r = 0.78 and 0.87, respectively) after marathon running (Moorthy & Zimmerman; Nieman, Berk, et al.). A negative correlation was also observed between training distance and degree of leukocytosis with the increase in cortisol ($r = -0.60$ for each) (Moorthy & Zimmerman). These data suggest that exercise-induced increases in serum cortisol and circulating leukocyte and granulocyte numbers are abrogated by longer or more intense training.

In contrast, other studies have failed to find a relationship between serum cortisol and leukocytosis occurring after exercise (Gimenez et al., 1986; Smith et al., 1989). Inconsistencies between studies may be explained by several factors, such as exercise intensity and duration and fitness level. Studies showing a relationship between cortisol and leukocytosis used intense endurance exercise, such as marathon running (Eskola et al., 1978; Moorthy & Zimmerman, 1978; Nieman, Berk, et al., 1989), whereas studies reporting no correlation have used shorter exercise in untrained or less fit subjects (Gimenez et al., 1986; Smith et al., 1989). Because serum cortisol levels may not always increase during brief exercise, it appears that cortisol contributes to leukocytosis (primarily via granulocytosis) only during intense prolonged exercise.

Exercise increases β-adrenergic activity, causing local release of norepinephrine, especially in blood vessels and the spleen, which may influence leukocyte migration as well as splenic output of cells. The tremendous increase in blood flow and opening of underperfused capillaries certainly contributes to the movement of leukocytes from the lungs into the vasculature (Muir et al., 1984). It does not appear that the spleen contributes much to exercise-induced leukocytosis (Hedfors, Biberfeld, & Wahren, 1978).

Exercise also profoundly changes leukocyte adrenergic receptors, which may influence their adherence to endothelial cells and thus migration patterns. Less than 10% of the increase in leukocyte number can be accounted for by exercise-induced hemoconcentration (Davidson et al., 1987; Ferry et al., 1990; McCarthy & Dale, 1988; Moorthy & Zimmerman, 1978; Priest et al., 1982). Acidosis caused by high lactate levels may influence mobilization of lymphocytes (Gimenez et al., 1986). Exercise may also stimulate bone marrow output of leukocytes via a delayed response, possibly via increases in factors such as IL-1 (McCarthy & Dale). However, the proportion of bone marrow–derived immature leukocytes to mature leukocytes does not appear to change during brief exercise (Christensen & Hill, 1987).

Model of Exercise-Induced Leukocytosis

The role of epinephrine and cortisol in exercise-induced leukocytosis has been extensively reviewed and a model proposed to explain leukocyte trafficking during and after exercise (McCarthy & Dale, 1988). McCarthy and Dale proposed that exercise-induced changes in leukocyte number and subset proportions can be explained by a combined effect of epinephrine and cortisol. Leukocytosis during brief exercise (less than 1 hr) is due to an increase in epinephrine. Because there is a lag in the appearance of cortisol in response to exercise, cortisol-induced increases in cell number occur 1 hr after the onset of exercise. During exercise lasting longer than 1 hr, the two hormones act simultaneously, and possibly synergistically, with maximum leukocytosis occurring 3 hr from the onset of exercise. At the end of exercise, the initial rapid decline in leukocyte number is due to rapid removal of epinephrine (within 30 min), whereas the prolonged elevation of leukocyte number is due to slower return of cortisol to baseline levels. During very prolonged exercise (or anytime during exercise in a fatigued athlete), depletion of catecholamines and cortisol may cause a decline in leukocyte number.

Effects of Exercise on Lymphocyte Proliferation

Lymphocytes are activated upon exposure to antigen entering the cell cycle and proliferating. This proliferation can be used as a functional measure of lymphocyte activation (Stites, 1987). The process can be assessed by an in vitro assay that measures incorporation of radioactively labeled precursors into lymphocyte DNA.

The effects of exercise on lymphocyte activation have been widely studied, using both human and experimental animal models. Various agents to stimulate lymphocyte proliferation have been used, including specific antigens or substances called mitogens because of their ability to stimulate mitosis (cell division) in lymphocytes. Mitogens used most often in exercise studies include concanavalin A (ConA), which stimulates T cell proliferation; phytohemmaglutinin (PHA), which stimulates a different subset of T cells to proliferate; pokeweed mitogen (PWM), a stimulator of T cell–dependent B cell proliferation; and lipopolysaccharide (LPS), which stimulates B cell proliferation in nonhuman species.

Human Lymphocyte Proliferative Response to Exercise

Response to T cell mitogens (ConA or PHA) may be suppressed by prolonged exercise (as shown in Figure 3.3), but the effect is transitory, with normal responsiveness restored 2 hr after exercise. For example, in runners, proliferative response to ConA stimulation

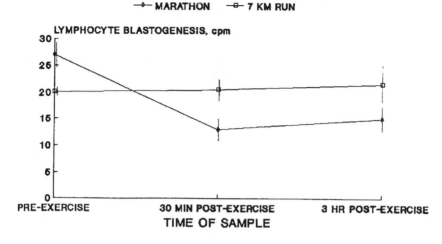

Figure 3.3 Lymphocyte proliferative response after exercise. Blood was obtained from marathon runners 30 min before and after and 3 hr after a marathon or a 7-km run. Heparanized blood was incubated with ConA in vitro and incorporation of ^{3}H-thymidine was measured after 72 hr. Bars represent SEM. Statistical significance not reported.

Note. From "Effect of Sport Stress on Lymphocyte Transformation and Antibody Formation" by J. Eskola, O. Ruuskanen, E. Soppi, M.K. Viljanen, M. Jarvinen, H. Toivonen, and K. Kouvalainen, 1978, *Clinical and Experimental Immunology*, **32**, p. 342. Copyright 1978 by Blackwell Scientific Publications. Adapted by permission.

decreased 50% following a marathon (Eskola et al., 1978; Gmunder et al., 1988). PHA response also decreased about 40% following marathon running (Eskola et al.) and cycling (Oshida et al., 1988; Tvede et al., 1989). Lymphocyte redistribution alone cannot account for suppression of mitogenic stimulation, because decreases in proliferative response to T cell mitogens may occur without changes in lymphocyte or T cell number (Eskola et al.; Gmunder et al.).

In contrast to prolonged exercise, shorter exercise (less than 1 hr) has little or no effect on T cell responsiveness to ConA and PHA (Edwards et al., 1984; Eskola et al., 1978; Hedfors et al., 1976; Robertson et al., 1981; Soppi et al., 1982). For example, in marathon runners, responses to ConA and PHA were unchanged 30 min after a 7-km run (Figure 3.3) (Eskola et al.). Untrained and trained individuals appear to show similar T cell responses to mitogenic challenge at rest and after moderate endurance exercise at the same relative exercise intensity (e.g., 2 hr of cycling at 60% $\dot{V}O_2$max) (Oshida et al., 1988).

Lymphocyte Proliferation in Animals

Studies on exercise-induced changes in human lymphocyte activation are limited by the availability of lymphoid cells that can be obtained (i.e., peripheral blood lymphocytes). Animal models can provide more complete data on cells from lymphoid tissues such as spleen, thymus, and lymph nodes. However, these studies are not without limitations. For example, forced exercise may introduce stress that may influence immune function.

Exhaustive exercise suppresses proliferative response to the T cell mitogen ConA in trained and untrained animals (Hoffman-Goetz, Keir, Thorne, & Houston, 1986; Mahan & Young, 1989; Simpson, Hoffman-Goetz, Thorne, & Arumugam, 1989). Suppression is most apparent in trained animals that are maximally exercised with less than 24 hr rest after the last training session (Hoffman-Goetz et al., 1986). The number of Ig-bearing B cells is also reduced by acute exhaustive exercise in untrained animals, suggesting suppression of T cell proliferation and subsequent stimulation of B cell differentiation (Simpson et al.). In untrained animals, reduced T cell responsiveness may be related to an exercise-induced increase in T_S cell number (Simpson et al.) as well as increased lymphocyte sensitivity to endogenous prostaglandin E_2 (PGE_2), a known suppressor of mitogenic response to ConA (Mahan & Young).

The suppressive effect of acute exhaustive exercise on T cell proliferation is abrogated by exercise training (see Figure 3.4). Trained animals also exhibit a lower percentage of splenic T_S cells in response to acute exhaustive exercise (Simpson et al., 1989). Moreover, exercise training reduces lymphocyte sensitivity to PGE_2 (Mahan & Young, 1989), suggesting less disturbance of T cell number and function in response to exhaustive exercise.

Exercise training also increased the number of T_H cells in several lymphoid organs (spleen, thymus, lymph nodes), but only in mice rested for 72 hr after the last exercise session (Hoffman-Goetz, Thorne, Randall-Simpson, & Arumugam, 1989). Responses to B cell mitogens (PWM and LPS) were also enhanced in trained but rested mice (Hoffman-Goetz, Thorne, & Houston, 1988), suggesting that regular moderate training may enhance T cell proliferative response and stimulation of B cell differentiation only if sufficient rest is provided.

Taken together, these data suggest that exhaustive exercise may impair T cell proliferation and subsequent stimulation of B cell differentiation. Exercise training appears to lessen or abolish this

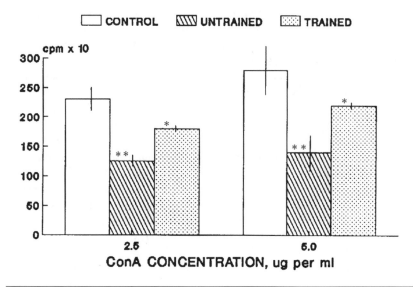

Figure 3.4   ConA response after exhaustive exercise. Untrained and trained rats swam to exhaustion (1-3 and 4-7 hr, respectively), and splenocyte proliferative responses to ConA stimulation were assayed by in vitro incorporation of ^{3}H-thymidine. Trained rats had swum 2 hr daily for 10 weeks prior to the exhaustive swim; untrained rats swam only the exhaustive swim; control rats performed neither training nor the exhaustive swim. Bars represent SEM. $*p < .05$, $**p < .01$ compared to control values.

Note. From "Immune Parameters of Untrained or Exercise Trained Rats After Exhaustive Exercise" by M.P. Mahan and M.R. Young, 1989, *Journal of Applied Physiology*, **66**, p. 284. Copyright 1989 by The American Physiological Society. Adapted by permission.

suppression, possibly by inducing less increase in T_S cell number or reducing sensitivity to PGE_2 or both. A lower glucocorticoid response to exercise may also be involved. Training may enhance T cell proliferation and B cell differentiation in well-rested animals.

Summary and Conclusions

Circulating leukocyte number increases markedly during exercise, and the magnitude of increase is related to exercise duration and intensity. The increase in leukocyte number is due primarily to an increase in granulocyte number. Exercise also increases circulating lymphocyte number and causes changes in the relative proportions of T, B, and NK cells as well as subsets of T cells (CD4 and CD8). After exercise, total leukocyte and granulocyte numbers may remain elevated for several hours, whereas lymphocyte number may decrease below baseline before returning to preexercise values.

The marked changes in leukocyte and lymphocyte numbers during exercise are transitory, and normal levels are restored within 24 hr. These changes reflect only redistribution of existing cells between different lymphoid compartments and do not indicate synthesis of new cells. That athletes exhibit normal resting cell counts and proliferative responses indicates that, over the long term, leukocyte function is relatively unaffected by exercise training. Whether the transitory effects of exercise on leukocyte function are related to susceptibility to illness is still open to speculation. Certainly physicians who treat athletes should be aware of possible perturbations in leukocyte counts that may persist for some time after exercise.

Chapter 4

Exercise and Innate Immunity: Phagocytes, Complement, and Acute Phase Proteins

I nnate immunity is usually the first aspect of immune function activated in response to an infectious agent. Innate immunity is mediated by a variety of structural and chemical barriers that limit entry into the host, as well as phagocytic cells that kill foreign microorganisms and release soluble factors that initiate the immune response.

Phagocytic Cells

Studies on exercise and phagocytes have focused on several parameters of phagocytic function that are measured in vitro, including cellular adherence, phagocytosis of particles, bactericidal activity, oxidative respiration, intracellular enzyme content, and cytotoxic and cytostatic activities. Cells from a variety of sources have been used to study phagocytic activity, such as peritoneal murine macrophages (Lotzerich, Fehr, & Appell, 1990), human connective tissue macrophages (Fehr, Lotzerich, & Michna, 1989), human peripheral blood monocytes and neutrophils (Busse et al., 1980; Lewicki et al., 1987; Smith, Telford, Mason, & Weidemann, 1990), and equine alveolar macrophages (Wong, Thompson, Thong, & Thornton, 1990). Phagocytic cells from different lymphoid tissues and from different species may not always respond similarly to exercise. Phagocytic functions may increase, decrease, or remain unchanged in response to a single bout of exercise, depending on the type of exercise and source of cells.

Macrophage Activity

Phagocytic activity of human connective tissue macrophages appears to be enhanced by exercise. For example, phagocytic activity, as measured by in vitro ingestion of latex beads, increased 30% to 60% following a 15-km exhaustive run in endurance-trained men (Fehr et al., 1989). Macrophage lysosomal enzyme content, measured histochemically, increased concomitantly. These studies suggest that macrophage phagocytic activity is enhanced following intense endurance exercise. However, it is unknown whether the response of this type of macrophage is representative of all pools of phagocytic cells. Work on monocytes/macrophages from other sources suggests that exercise does not always enhance macrophage function (Bieger et al., 1980; Wong et al., 1990). For example, phagocytic activity decreased in blood monocytes following brief maximal running (Bieger et al.).

Antibacterial activity of alveolar macrophages is important in resistance to lower respiratory illness in horses, common in animals subjected to stress and exercise (Wong et al., 1990). Alveolar macrophage microbicidal activity, measured by chemiluminescence, decreased 50% within 30 min after exercise, remained low for 3 days, and returned to normal by 5 days after exercise. There were no changes in the types or numbers of cells obtained from the lung, indicating that changes in total activity were due to a decrease in macrophage killing activity. These data may indicate impaired macrophage antibacterial activity following intense exercise in horses. Because these horses were previously untrained, the response to exercise cannot be distinguished from the response to stress of a novel situation (i.e., treadmill running). It is also unknown whether macrophage activity is normalized after adjusting to strenuous exercise training.

In addition to their phagocytic and secretory functions, macrophages exhibit antitumor activity, which can be divided into cytotoxic (killing) and cytostatic (growth-inhibitory) activities. Peritoneal murine macrophages, isolated from untrained mice run to exhaustion on a treadmill, exhibited enhanced cytostatic but not cytotoxic activity against tumor cells in an in vitro assay (Lotzerich et al., 1990). Binding of macrophages to tumor cells was unchanged after exercise. Although limited, these data suggest that exercise may enhance macrophage secretion of a soluble factor, possibly TNF, that inhibits tumor cell growth without influencing macrophage binding and killing activity.

Neutrophil Activity

Neutrophil microbicidal activity appears to be either enhanced (Smith, Telford, Mason, & Weidemann, 1990) or unchanged (Busse et al., 1980) following moderate exercise. For example, oxidative activity was measured in neutrophils exposed to coated particles in an in vitro system (Smith, Telford, Mason, & Weidemann); upon ingestion of the particles, neutrophil oxidative activity increased. In both trained and untrained subjects neutrophil oxidative activity increased and remained elevated for 6 hr following exercise (1 hr cycling at 60% $\dot{V}O_2$max) (Figure 4.1). However, responses of specific parameters of neutrophil oxidative activity differed between trained and untrained subjects. Postexercise oxidative activity at low particle concentration was lower in athletes than nonathletes, suggesting a lower affinity of neutrophils for particles in trained athletes. These data may indicate reduced neutrophil responsiveness in athletes compared to untrained individuals.

Running has also been associated with increased activation of neutrophils. Release of polymorphonuclear elastase, an indicator of

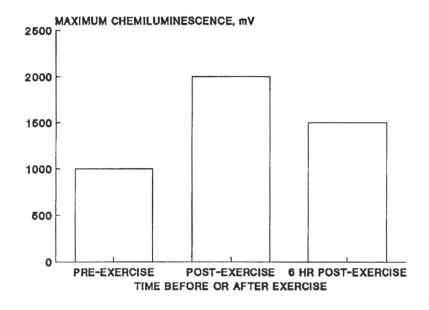

Figure 4.1 Neutrophil activation after exercise. A typical individual response of reactive oxygen production in human neutrophils stimulated with zymosan particles. Statistical significance of individual data not reported.

Note. From "Exercise, Training and Neutrophil Microbicidal Activity" by J.A. Smith, R.D. Telford, I.B. Mason, and M.J. Weidemann, 1990, International Journal of Sports Medicine, 11, p. 181. Copyright 1990 by Georg Thieme Verlag. Adapted by permission.

neutrophil activation, increased following 2-km and 10-km runs, with higher release after the longer run (Schaefer, Kokot, Heidland, & Plass, 1987). Smith, Telford, Mason, and Weidemann (1990) suggested that the increase in neutrophil activity following exercise may be due to stimulation by cytokines released during exercise, such as IL-1, IL-2, TNFα, or GM-CSF, or various hormones such as epinephrine or β-endorphin. Alternatively, increased neutrophil activity may be due to redistribution of neutrophils, which may bring into the circulation a more active subset of neutrophil. However, Smith, Telford, Mason, and Weidemann discounted this possibility, based on their data showing no association between neutrophil distribution and oxidative activity following other forms of exercise.

The increase in neutrophil oxidative activity observed in both trained and untrained subjects suggests an enhancement of neutrophil microbicidal activity following moderate exercise (Smith, Telford, Mason, & Weidemann, 1990). In contrast, microbicidal activity as measured by the number of killed ingested bacteria in an in vitro assay did not change after shorter (30 min) maximal exercise in both cyclists and nonathletes (Lewicki et al., 1987). Neutrophils from cyclists exhibited significantly lower microbicidal activity both at rest and after exercise compared to cells from nonathletes.

Taken together, the data from these studies suggest that neutrophil microbicidal activity increases following moderate exercise regardless of training status and that neutrophil activity appears unchanged by brief strenuous exercise. However, neutrophil activity appears to be lower in trained athletes both at rest and following moderate and intense exercise than in nonathletes. It has been suggested that in athletes partial suppression of neutrophil activity may act to reduce the inflammatory response to low-level tissue damage (Smith, Telford, Mason, & Weidemann, 1990), which may occur during regular training. It is unclear if this apparent chronic suppression of neutrophil function occurs in other types of athletes, or whether it alters nonspecific immunity in elite athletes.

Complement

Only a few studies have looked at serum complement levels in response to exercise. Total complement titer, as measured in a functional assay, was reported to increase 14% following a single 20-min bout of intense cycling in nonathletes but remained unchanged following 2 weeks of heavy weight training in experienced resistance athletes (Eberhardt, 1971). Neither study corrected for possible changes in plasma volumes following acute exercise or training.

Complement components C3 and C4 remained unchanged after 1 hr of running (Hanson & Flaherty, 1981) but increased slightly (11%-15%) following a brief graded maximal run (Figure 4.2) (Nieman, Tan, Lee, & Berk, 1989). C3 and C4 levels were lower at rest and after maximal running in marathon runners than in untrained control subjects (Nieman, Tan, et al.). No correlations were observed between training distance and resting C3 or C4 levels. The pattern of increased complement levels after exercise and lower absolute levels in athletes compared to nonathletes is similar to that observed for acute phase proteins (see later discussion). It has been suggested that this represents long-term adaptation to chronic inflammation resulting from daily intense exercise in athletes. Although resting and postexercise complement levels were lower in athletes, these values were still within the clinically normal range (Nieman, Tan, et al.).

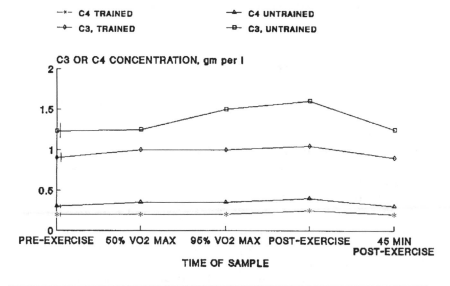

Figure 4.2 Serum complement in athletes and nonathletes. Serum C3 and C4 levels were measured in trained and untrained individuals before, during, and after a maximum graded exercise test. Bars represent SEM for baseline values. $p < .05$ for C4 levels, athletes versus controls, at rest, during exercise, and during recovery; $p < .01$ for C3 levels, athletes versus controls at rest, during exercise, and during recovery; $p < .01$ for preexercise versus recovery C3 and C4 levels for each group.

Note. From "Complement and Immunoglobulin Levels in Athletes and Sedentary Controls" by D.C. Nieman, S.A. Tan, J.W. Lee, and L.S. Berk, 1989, *International Journal of Sports Medicine*, **10**, p. 126. Copyright 1989 by Georg Thieme Verlag. Adapted by permission.

Complement C3a and C4a fragments were significantly elevated after 2.5 hr intense running in athletes, and C4a remained elevated for 3 hr after the run (Dufaux & Order, 1989). It was suggested that increases in these complement cleavage fragments indicate complement activation by both the classical and alternative pathways during exercise and that complement activation may be involved in clearance of damaged tissue after intense prolonged exercise.

In contrast, no changes in serum C3 concentration were noted after 2 hr uphill walking at 40% $\dot{V}O_2$max in the heat, although C3 level was higher during and after exercise in the hypohydrated compared to the euhydrated state (Sawka et al., 1989). When intravascular C3 mass was calculated to adjust for changes in plasma volume, there were no differences between the two conditions. These data indicate that dehydration itself can influence plasma complement concentration without appreciable changes in the absolute amount of complement.

Acute Phase Proteins

Acute phase proteins (APP), glycoprotein molecules found in serum during acute infection or inflammation, increase following intense endurance exercise (Dufaux, Order, Geyer, & Hollmann, 1984; Liesen, Dufaux, & Hollmann, 1977). For example, the concentration of serum C-reactive protein (CRP), the major APP, increased 6-fold following 2 and 3 hr of running and remained elevated for up to 3 days after each run (Figure 4.3) (Liesen et al.). CRP levels were higher after 2 hr of high-intensity running compared with low-intensity running of the same duration. However, the highest CRP levels were recorded after a 3-hr run at the lower intensity, suggesting that postexercise serum CRP levels reflect combined effects of both intensity and duration. Other APP, such as protease inhibitors and iron-binding proteins, are also elevated after endurance running, and some may remain elevated for up to 6 days (Liesen et al.).

Resting levels of CRP are lower in some types of athletes compared to nonathletes (Dufaux et al., 1984). For example, swimmers and rowers exhibited lower resting CRP levels than middle- and long-distance runners, road cyclists, and soccer players, who showed CRP levels similar to untrained control subjects (Dufaux et al.).

Dufaux et al. (1984) suggested that the lower CRP levels in swimmers and rowers could be attributed to lower mechanical stress on the body as a result of these activities compared to others. However,

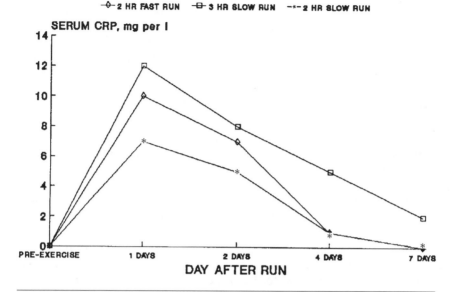

Figure 4.3 Serum C-reactive protein (CRP) after running. Serum CRP was measured in runners after 2- and 3-hr runs. Slow runs were at 65% to 85% of the running speed at onset of blood lactate accumulation (OBLA), assumed to be 4 mmol · l^{-1}; fast runs were at 82% to 95% of speed at OBLA. Standard errors and statistical significance not reported.

Note. From "Modifications of Serum Glycoproteins the Days Following a Prolonged Physical Exercise and the Influence of Physical Training" by H. Liesen, B. Dufaux, and W. Hollmann, 1977, *European Journal of Applied Physiology*, **37**, p. 245. Copyright 1977 by Springer-Verlag. Adapted by permission.

this cannot completely explain the lower CRP levels in swimmers and rowers compared to nonathletes. A dual effect of exercise training was suggested: an acute effect of a single exercise session that elevates CRP for up to 3 days and chronic suppression of CRP due to continued high intensity training. Thus, because swimming and rowing induce less mechanical stress, the chronic effect (suppression of APP) predominates, resulting in low CRP levels. Athletes in more mechanically stressful sports would exhibit both acute and chronic effects, with the end result of normal CRP levels.

Earlier data from the same laboratory support the concept of chronic suppression of APP following exercise training (Liesen et al., 1977). For example, postexercise (2 hr of running) CRP levels were lower after 9 weeks of endurance training than before training, despite a higher running velocity after training. Similar trends were seen for other APP, such as haptoglobin and α-1-acid glycoprotein. In contrast, resting serum levels of some protease inhibitors were higher in well-trained athletes than in nonathletes (Liesen et al.). Higher activity of protease inhibitors may limit proteolytic activity in muscle and connective tissue after exercise.

The significance of these changes in serum APP, especially with regard to immune function, is not clear. APP are released in response to infection as well as inflammation or injury, such as that induced by intense prolonged exercise. It is not clear if elevated APP observed after exercise indicates an enhanced ability to respond to bacterial infection, or whether lower resting levels of APP observed in some athletes indicate suppression of innate immunity. If low levels of APP influence immune reactivity, then it follows that athletes with the lowest APP levels, such as swimmers and rowers, should exhibit the highest rates of infection. This, though, has not yet been documented. APP release is stimulated by some cytokines, such as IL-1, IL-6, and TNFα, which have been shown to increase during exercise. The role of these substances in inflammation resulting from exercise training is currently unknown.

Summary and Conclusions

Innate immunity represents diverse functions of the early immune response to infectious agents and some types of tumor cells. The effects of exercise on parameters of innate immunity have not been thoroughly explored. The few recently published studies suggest that, in humans, neutrophil and macrophage phagocytotic activity may be enhanced immediately following moderate and possibly intense endurance exercise. However, these responses may be lower in elite endurance athletes than in nonathletes. Similarly, serum complement and acute phase proteins increase following exercise but are lower at rest and after exercise in well-trained athletes than in nonathletes. This apparent suppression may represent adjustments to chronic inflammation resulting from intense training. The implications of these changes for resistance to infection are unknown at this point, and further work is needed to determine if exercise influences the innate immune response to infection.

Chapter 5

Exercise and Humoral Immunity: Immunoglobulin, Antibody, and Mucosal Immunity

A ntibody is an important effector of host resistance to infectious agents, and production of antibody is a major feature of acquired immunity ("memory"). High levels of immunoglobulins (Ig) and antibodies are found in serum and mucosal fluids, such as tears, saliva, and secretions of the genito-urinary, respiratory, and gastrointestinal tracts. Levels of Ig and specific antibodies differ between serum and mucosal fluids. The responses of Ig and antibodies in these fluids to immunogenic challenge are not necessarily related.

Serum Immunoglobulins

IgG (the predominant Ig in serum), IgA, and IgM were reported to be within clinically normal levels in male marathon runners at rest (Green et al., 1981; Nieman, Tan, et al., 1989). In contrast, in elite distance runners serum IgG concentration was reported to be higher early in the training season compared to nonathlete control subjects (Wit, 1984). Resting serum IgG decreased during the season, reaching its lowest level during major competition; however, the lowest IgG concentration was still well within the range observed in the control subjects. Serum IgA and IgM also exhibited similar patterns throughout the season; IgM levels were always within the normal range, whereas serum IgA was either at the low end or below normal levels.

Ig Response to Exercise

Intense exercise during regular training does not appear to alter serum Ig levels as measured by total serum IgG, IgA, IgM, or IgE concentration or intravascular mass. For example, in trained runners, serum levels of IgG, IgA, IgM, and IgE were unchanged immediately and 24 hr after a normal 13-km training run (Hanson & Flaherty, 1981). Serum IgA, IgG, and IgM concentrations were also unchanged after 2 hours of intense cycling (Mackinnon, Chick, van As, & Tomasi, 1989) and after a brief maximal exercise test in both athletes and nonathletes (Nieman, Tan, et al., 1989). Moreover, when adjusted for changes in plasma volume, intravascular masses of IgG, IgA, and IgM were noted to be unchanged after 45 min of walking in a hot (35 °C) environment (Sawka et al., 1989).

In contrast to serum levels of Ig, production of Ig in vitro may be reduced after exercise. For example, in vitro production of IgG, IgA, and IgM was lower in lymphocytes from untrained subjects after 15 min of moderate cycling than in cells obtained before exercise; this effect was seen in both unstimulated and PWM-stimulated cells (Hedfors et al., 1983). The largest reduction was seen in IgA production. In this study, exercise also caused a redistribution of circulating lymphocytes, notably a 30% reduction in the percent of T_H (CD4) cells. Because T_H cells are essential to B cell differentiation and Ig synthesis, the reduction in Ig production in vitro could be accounted for by a transitory change in lymphocyte subsets at the time of sampling. That is, the capacity for B cells to produce Ig may be maintained, but fewer T_H cells may provide less stimulation of Ig production. Because lymphocyte subset distribution is restored after exercise, measuring the in vitro response may not accurately reflect the effects of exercise on Ig production in the body.

Antibodies to Specific Antigens

Exercise training may enhance specific antibody formation in response to immunogenic challenge. For example, in male runners a slightly higher titer of serum Ig specific to injected tetanus toxoid was observed after a 42-km marathon compared to nonathletes injected at the same time (Eskola et al., 1978). In an experimental animal model, when mice were trained to run on a treadmill for several weeks prior to immunization with injected *Salmonella typhi*, the exercised mice exhibited markedly higher specific antibody to the bacteria than did nontrained control mice immunized at the same time (Figure 5.1) (Liu & Wang, 1986/87).

A reduction in total Ig concentration has been observed in some athletes during intense training before and during major competition (Kassil, Levando, Suzdal'nitskii, Pershin, & Kuz'min, 1988;

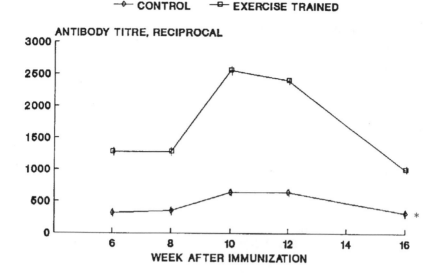

Figure 5.1 Serum antibodies to *Salmonella typhi* in exercised mice. Exercise-trained mice were run daily for 23 days prior to infection with *Salmonella typhi* and continued training after infection. Control mice were infected at the same time but never exercised. Bars represent 2 × SEM. *p < .05 exercised versus control mice.

Note. From "The Enhancing Effect of Exercise on the Production of Antibody to *Salmonella Typhi* in Mice" by Y.G. Liu and S.Y. Wang, 1986/87, *Immunology Letters*, **14**, p. 119. Copyright 1987 by Elsevier Science Publishers. Adapted by permission.

Pershin, Kuz'min, Suzdal'nitskii, & Levando, 1988; Wit, 1984), and these changes may also reflect changes in specific antibodies. For example, in Soviet sportsmen (sports unspecified) serum antibodies to tetanus, diptheria, and staphylococcus decreased during major competition, although these antibodies were unchanged by intense training alone (Figure 5.2) (Pershin et al.).

These limited data, together with studies of resting Ig levels discussed above, suggest that intense exercise does not by itself alter serum Ig and may increase specific antibodies. However, it is possible that the combination of intense training and the psychological stress of competition may alter both total Ig and specific antibody levels. It is currently unclear whether these changes are of clinical significance.

Mechanisms of Changes in Ig

It is to be expected that serum Ig levels are unchanged after a single bout of exercise, because circulating Ig is a function of B and plasma

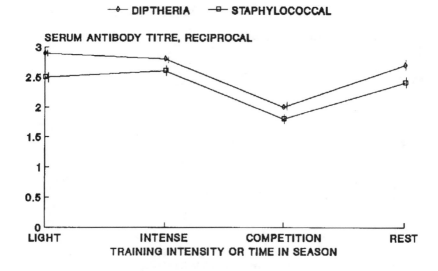

Figure 5.2 Specific antibodies throughout the training season. Normally occurring serum antibodies specific to diptheria and staphylococcus were measured in sportsmen at various times in the training season. Bars represent SEM. Statistical significance not reported.
Note. From "Reserve Potential of Immunity" by B.B. Pershin, S.N. Kuz'min, R.S. Suzdal'nitskii, and V.A. Levando, 1988, *Sports Training, Medicine and Rehabilitation,* **1,** p. 55. Copyright 1988 by Harwood Academic Publishers. Adapted by permission.

cell secretion. Ig production by these cells generally does not change over the short term. The observation that resting serum Ig levels are normal in athletes also suggests that, over the long term, baseline Ig production is not affected by exercise. The higher specific antibody response observed after acute exercise and training is unexplained at present, but it may represent an enhanced capacity of the immune system to respond to antigenic challenge. Factors possibly involved include cytokines, such as the interleukins, which are important to B cell proliferation and differentiation. Alternatively, the process of antigen presentation or T cell recognition or both may also be enhanced following exercise.

Mucosal Immunoglobulins

IgA, the predominant Ig in mucosal fluids, is a major effector of host defense against microorganisms causing illnesses such as URI

(Tomasi & Plaut, 1985). IgA helps prevent URI via inhibition of viral and bacterial attachment to the mucosal epithelium, as well as viral replication.

The high incidence of URI among elite athletes, especially during intense training and major competition, has prompted studies on the effects of exercise on secretory IgA. Exercise-induced decreases in IgA levels in oral and nasal fluids could in theory provide a mechanism for the apparent susceptibility of these athletes to URI. In addition, psychological stress is associated with increased rate of URI (Graham, Douglas, & Ryan, 1986) and decreased secretory IgA levels (Jemmott et al., 1983), suggesting that the psychological stress of major competition may play a role in altering IgA levels and resistance to URI.

Exercise-induced decreases in salivary and nasal wash IgA levels have been reported in a variety of competitive athletes, including Nordic skiers (Tomasi et al., 1982), cyclists (Mackinnon et al., 1989), swimmers (Tharp & Barnes, 1990), runners (Muns, Liesen, Riedel, & Bergmann, 1989), hockey players, squash athletes, and kayakers (Mackinnon, Ginn, & Seymour, in press), and a variety of Soviet sportspeople (unspecified sports; Levando, Suzdal'nitskii, Pershin, & Zykov, 1988).

The first study to document changes in IgA levels (Tomasi et al., 1982) reported that male and female members of the U.S. National Nordic ski team exhibited lower resting salivary IgA concentration than age-matched control subjects. IgA level decreased 40% following 2- to 3-hr races during the National Championship. It was suggested that the low resting IgA concentration may be due to chronic suppression resulting from daily intense training and possibly to psychological stress preceding major competition. It was also noted that the lower IgA levels after the race could be due to a combination of factors, such as intense exercise, cold ambient temperature, or competition stress.

Subsequent work from the same lab confirmed that stimulated salivary IgA levels decrease after intense endurance exercise in the controlled environment and a noncompetitive laboratory setting (Mackinnon et al., 1989). Competitive cyclists pedaled for 2 hr at 90% of ventilatory threshold (70% to 80% $\dot{V}O_2$max). IgA concentration, corrected for changes in salivary protein, was 60% lower immediately after exercise, remained low for 1 hr, and returned to preexercise levels by 24 hr after the single exercise session. IgM, a minor mucosal Ig, also exhibited the same trend, whereas IgG concentration remained unchanged, indicating a specific effect on mucosal Ig.

In a study on university swimmers over a 4-month season, IgA concentration decreased about 10% following each of four training sessions lasting 2 hr each (Figure 5.3) (Tharp & Barnes, 1990). Both resting and postexercise IgA levels declined progressively (about 25%) over the season, as training intensity increased from light to heavy. During the taper period IgA levels appeared to recover partially toward early season levels, and they did not decline as much after exercise compared to earlier training sessions. These data suggest that the cumulative effects of intense daily training may have a more pronounced effect on IgA levels than a single exercise session.

At any given time, salivary IgA concentration appears to be a function of several factors, including these (Mackinnon et al., 1990; Muns et al., 1989; Tharp & Barnes, 1990; Tomasi et al., 1982):

- Intensity of the exercise session
- The preceding training period
- Psychological stress associated with training and competing at the elite level

In runners, salivary IgA levels were reported to decrease 40% and to remain low for 18 hr following a 31-km race (Muns et al.).

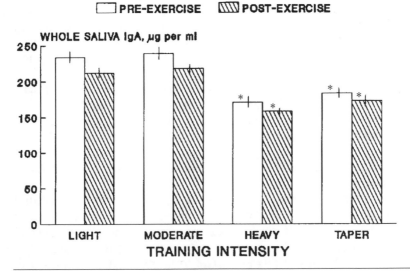

Figure 5.3 Salivary IgA response to swim training. Whole salivary IgA concentration, expressed as µg IgA per ml saliva, was measured in collegiate swimmers before and after usual training at various times in the season. Bars represent SEM. $*p < .05$ compared to light and moderate training intensity.

Note. From "Reduction of Saliva Immunoglobulin Levels by Swim Training" by G.D. Tharp and M.W. Barnes, 1990, *European Journal of Applied Physiology*, **60**, p. 62. Copyright 1990 by Springer-Verlag. Adapted by permission.

Prolonged recovery of mucosal IgA levels following intense exercise may have implications for elite athletes who train at least once daily.

It has been suggested that in some athletes mucosal IgA levels may be related more to psychological stress of major competition than to exercise per se (Mackinnon et al., 1990). For example, in female hockey athletes, resting and postexercise IgA and IgM concentrations were lower during major competition than during training before competition (Mackinnon et al.). In addition, resting and postexercise IgA concentrations were reduced by a week of purposefully intense training in elite male kayakers (Mackinnon, Ginn, & Seymour, in press). In this study, IgA flow rate (the rate of IgA appearance in saliva) decreased 27% to 51% following each of four kayak training sessions (Figure 5.4). The largest decrease was observed during the session at the end of an intense week of training.

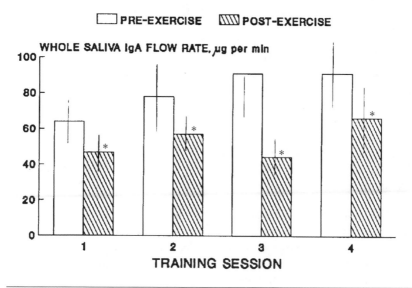

Figure 5.4 Salivary IgA flow rates after kayak training. Whole salivary IgA flow rate, expressed as μg IgA per minute, was measured before and after usual training during four training sessions in elite male kayakers. Session 3 was an especially intense session at the end of a week of hard training. Bars represent SEM. *$p < .02$, compared to preexercise values.
Note. Reprinted with permission from "Effects of Exercise During Sports Training and Competition on Salivary IgA Levels" by L.T. Mackinnon, E. Ginn, and G. Seymour. In *Behaviour and Immunity: Proceedings of the 1990 Australian Behavioural Immunology Group Scientific Meeting* edited by A. Husband (in press). Copyright CRC Press, Inc., Boca Raton, FL. Adapted by permission.

Taken together, these data indicate that the total amount of IgA on the oral mucosal surface (a function of both IgA flow rate and IgA concentration) are reduced following a single session of intense endurance exercise. There also appears to be a cumulative effect of intense daily training on pre- and postexercise IgA concentration and flow rate, as well as on the magnitude of change from before to after exercise. In addition, psychological stress associated with intense training and major competition appears to interact with exercise in altering mucosal antibody levels.

Are Exercise-Induced Changes in IgA Related to URI?

Although intense exercise is associated with a high incidence of URI and decreased secretory IgA levels, a causal relationship has not been clearly established. However, preliminary data from two groups of elite athletes studied over an extended period suggest a temporal relationship between exercise-induced decreases in salivary IgA concentration and appearance of URI (Mackinnon, Ginn, & Seymour, 1991b). Elite squash and hockey athletes were studied, with saliva samples collected before and after usual training, weekly over 10 weeks for squash athletes, and daily over 10 days for hockey athletes. Five of 14 squash athletes (36%) and 5 of 19 hockey athletes (26%) exhibited URI, as documented by the team physicians; no other illnesses were reported. In squash athletes, six of the seven episodes of illness were preceded within 2 days by a 22% decrease in IgA levels following the usual workout. Similarly, in hockey athletes, all five episodes of URI were preceded within 2 days by a 23% decrease in IgA levels. In contrast, IgA remained unchanged or increased slightly in athletes who did not develop illness.

Mechanisms Decreasing Mucosal IgA

The mechanism or mechanisms responsible for decreased mucosal IgA following intense exercise are unclear at present but may involve changes in migration of plasma cells or local secretion of IgA or both (Mackinnon et al., 1989). Circulatory changes during exercise may alter migration of IgA-secreting plasma cells to the oral mucosa. Alternatively, exercise may reduce plasma cell secretion of IgA or transport of IgA across the epithelial cell barrier. These possibilities have yet to be explored.

Reduction of IgA levels only in elite athletes during intense exercise and during times of stress strongly suggests a neuroendocrine component. However, neither mood state nor salivary cortisol levels were reportedly correlated with changes in salivary IgA during intense training; it was suggested that the profile mood state may not have been sufficiently sensitive to measure changes over time (Tharp & Barnes, 1990). The possible role of other neuroendocrine factors in regulation of mucosal immunity in athletes has not been pursued.

Summary and Conclusions

Resting serum Ig levels are clinically normal and do not appear to change with exercise. Resting Ig and specific antibody levels may be reduced during intense sport training in elite athletes but are restored by reduced training after the season ends. Serum antibodies to specific pathogens may be increased following acute exercise or exercise training. In elite athletes, resting and postexercise secretory IgA levels decrease during heavy training and are partially restored during the taper (reduced training loads). Secretory IgA decreases after intense prolonged exercise, especially in competitive athletes.

Transitory changes in IgA after exercise appear to be temporally related to the appearance of upper respiratory illness in elite athletes. However, even after intense exercise, athletes are not clinically IgA-deficient. Although exercise-induced changes in IgA levels may explain part of the increased susceptibility of athletes to upper respiratory illness, it is likely that additional factors are involved.

Chapter 6

Exercise and Cytokines: Interleukins, Interferon, and Tumor Necrosis Factor

Soluble factors such as cytokines are important in initiating and regulating the immune response, influencing virtually all immune functions. As detailed in chapter 2, cytokines are primarily growth factors, stimulating proliferation and differentiation of various immune cells as well as other types of cells (e.g., fibroblasts). Considering the central role of cytokines in immune regulation, it is surprising that there are few published studies on the effects of exercise on these substances (see Table 6.1); certainly this is one exciting area for further work.

Interleukin-1

IL-1 was the first lymphokine to be studied in the exercise literature (Cannon, Evans, Hughes, Meredith, & Dinarello, 1986; Cannon & Kluger, 1983). IL-1 activity was higher compared to resting levels in plasma taken from subjects immediately and 3 hr after cycling for 1 hr at 60% $\dot{V}O_2$max (Cannon & Kluger). A later study using a more sensitive bioassay reported that IL-1 activity did not increase immediately after but was elevated by 50% for 3 to 6 hr after exercise, returning to baseline values by 9 hr of recovery (Cannon et al.). The increase in IL-1 activity measured in vitro was inhibited by anti-IL-1 antibodies, indicating a specific effect due to IL-1 and not other factors such as IL-2.

Resting IL-1 levels have been reported to be higher in endurance runners than nonathletes, and the IL-1 response to exercise may differ between athletes and nonathletes (Evans et al., 1986). For example, in untrained subjects IL-1 activity increased 3 hr after moderate eccentric exercise (27%-42% $\dot{V}O_2$max) sufficient to cause

Table 6.1   Summary of Exercise and Cytokines

Cytokine	Major effects	Response to exercise
IL-1	Induces fever IL-2 release IL-2r expression IL-6 release APP (CRP) release	Increases after 1 hr of moderate exercise Higher at rest in runners
IL-2	IL-2r expression T cell activation NK cell activation	Decreased IL-2 production Decreased IL-2 level Increased IL-2 level 24 hr after running
IL-6	T and B cell activation APP release	Increased after running
IFNα	Antiviral activity NK cell activation Antitumor activity Induces fever	Increased after moderate exercise
TNFα	Antitumor activity Induces fever Cachexia Antiviral activity	Increased after running Increased after moderate exercise in untrained

Note. Moderate exercise = 50%-70% $\dot{V}O_2$max.

Data from Cannon, Evans, Hughes, Meredith, and Dinarello (1986); Espersen, Elbaek, Ernst, Toft, Kaalund, Jersild, and Grunnet (1990); Flegel, Mannel, Baumstark, Berg, and Northoff (1989); Haahr, Pedersen, Fomsgaard, Tvede, Diamant, Klarlund, Halkjaer-Kristensen, and Bendtzen (in press); Lewicki, Tchorzewski, Majewska, Nowak, and Baj (1988); Smith Telford, Baker, Hapel, and Weidemann (1990); Viti, Muscettola, Paulesu, Bocci, and Almi (1985).

muscle soreness; in contrast, IL-1 activity increased slightly or decreased in four runners after the same exercise. For both groups IL-1 activity returned to preexercise levels by 24 hr after exercise.

Because the runners had refrained from training for only 2 days prior to testing, it was unclear whether the higher resting IL-1 levels were related to a training effect or to the last training session (Evans et al., 1986). Elevated resting IL-1 is unlikely to be a long-lasting acute effect of exercise because normal IL-1 levels are restored by 9 to 24 hr after exercise (Cannon et al., 1986; Evans et al.). An elevated resting IL-1 level in runners is consistent with high resting serum levels of CRP (Dufaux et al., 1984) and creatine kinase (Evans et al.); these changes may reflect chronic inflammation, muscle damage, or both resulting from intense daily training. It was suggested that high resting IL-1 levels in runners reflect muscle proteolysis and repair as a result of intense regular exercise (Evans et al.).

In vitro production of IL-1 also appears to be elevated following exercise (Cannon & Kluger, 1983; Haahr et al., in press; Lewicki et al., 1988). For example, adherent cells (primarily monocytes) isolated from cyclists immediately after exercise exhibited a 78% increase in IL-1 production; a further increase in IL-1 production was noted in cells obtained 2 hr after the exercise test (Figure 6.1) (Lewicki et al., 1988). Because a constant number of adherent cells was used in the assays, it is likely that the increase in IL-1 concentration reflects enhanced IL-1 production. Elevated in vitro

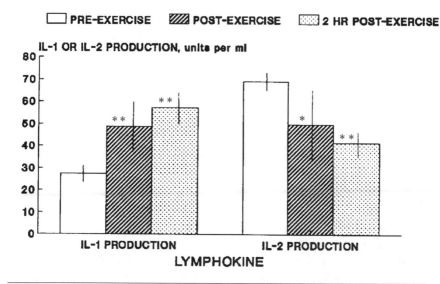

Figure 6.1   IL-1 and IL-2 production after exercise. In vitro IL-1 and IL-2 production were measured in peripheral blood mononuclear cells (adherent and nonadherent, respectively) cultured for 48 hr in the presence of mitogens (LPS for IL-1 and PHA for IL-2). Bars represent SEM. *$p < .05$; **$p < .01$ compared to preexercise values.

Note. From "Effect of Maximal Physical Exercise on T-Lymphocyte Subpopulations and on Interleukin-1 (IL 1) and Interleukin-2 (IL 2) Production in Vitro" by R. Lewicki, H. Tchorzewski, E. Majewska, A. Nowak, and Z. Baj, 1988, *International Journal of Sports Medicine,* **9**, p. 116. Copyright 1988 by Georg Thieme Verlag. Adapted by permission.

production of IL-1 is consistent with increased levels in the plasma observed after exercise (Cannon et al., 1986), suggesting that monocyte production of IL-1 is stimulated by exercise.

It is not yet clear whether higher levels of IL-1 observed at rest in athletes and after exercise in both athletes and nonathletes are related to changes in immune function. Increases in circulating IL-1 levels may stimulate lymphocyte proliferation, although this appears unlikely for several reasons: First, increases in lymphocyte proliferation have not been noted following exercise similar to that reported to increase IL-1 levels (Eskola et al., 1978; Tvede et al., 1989), and lymphocyte proliferation may be impaired after more intense exercise (see chapter 3) (Eskola et al.; Gmunder et al., 1988). Second, resting lymphocyte proliferation and cell numbers are similar in athletes and nonathletes (Oshida et al., 1988). Third, increases in IL-1 do not appear to stimulate IL-2 production after exercise (see later discussion); IL-1 stimulation of IL-2 production is important to initiating lympocyte proliferation.

It is possible that the stimulatory effects of increases in IL-1 levels are offset by a decrease in the $T_H:T_S$ ratio or increases in substances that oppose IL-1 (Cannon et al., 1986). Exercise-induced increases in IL-1 level may be related to augmentation of cytotoxic activity observed after some types of exercise (see chapter 7). Increases in IL-1 levels may also underly increases in TNFα and IL-6 after exercise (see later discussion) (Flegel, Mannel, Baumstark, Berg, & Northoff, 1989; Smith, Telford, Baker, Hapel, & Weidemann, 1990).

Interleukin-2

IL-2 levels in plasma and in vitro IL-2 production are reduced following exercise (Espersen et al., 1990; Lewicki et al., 1988; Pahlavani, Cheung, Chesky, & Richardson, 1988). For example, in trained runners, plasma IL-2 concentration decreased 50% immediately after a 5-km race, returned to baseline levels by 2 hr after, and then increased by 50% 24 hr after the race (Espersen et al., 1990). It was suggested that the transitory decrease in IL-2 level immediately after exercise may reflect a concomitant increase in the number of activated lymphocytes expressing the IL-2 receptor (i.e., more cells with more receptors removing IL-2 from the circulation; Espersen et al., 1990). The delayed increase in IL-2 level observed 24 hr after exercise could not be accounted for by changes in lymphocyte number or distribution and may reflect postrace inflammation stimulating release of lymphokines such as IL-1 or IL-2.

In trained cyclists, in vitro IL-2 production was reduced 27% in lymphocytes obtained immediately after a 20-min incremental cycling test to $\dot{V}O_2$max; IL-2 production was 40% lower 2 hr after exercise compared to before (Figure 6.1) (Lewicki et al., 1988). The decrease in IL-2 production may have been related to a 30% decrease in T_H cell number, with a corresponding decline in the $T_H:T_S$ ratio.

The decline in IL-2 production following brief maximal exercise may indicate a reduced ability of lymphoyctes to respond to immunogenic challenge. However, lymphocyte proliferation appears to be unaffected by this level of exercise (see chapter 3). It is unknown whether prolonged exercise influences IL-2 production or whether changes in IL-2 levels are related to decreases in lymphocyte responsiveness observed after prolonged exercise (Eskola et al., 1978; Gmunder et al., 1988).

Exercise and the IL-2 Receptor

Expression of the IL-2 receptor (IL-2r) may be augmented or decreased following exercise, depending on the assay system (Lewicki et al., 1988). A 3-fold increase in the percentage of cells exhibiting the Tac antigen (IL-2r) was observed in nonstimulated lymphocytes isolated from cyclists after 20 min of maximal exercise; the increase in IL-2r positive cells was maintained for 2 hr after exercise. On the other hand, when cells were stimulated in vitro with PHA, IL-2r expression was lower in cells obtained at both times after exercise compared to before.

The increase in the relatively small percentage (less than 5%) of nonstimulated cells expressing the IL-2r may reflect changes in circulating subsets of T cells. Resting T cells do not normally exhibit large numbers of the IL-2r subunit recognized by the anti-Tac monoclonal antibody. Activation of T cells increases expression of this subunit (Roitt et al., 1989); thus the lower number of PHA-stimulated cells exhibiting the IL-2r after exercise may be a better indicator of the effect of exercise on IL-2r expression. Again, it is unclear whether exercise-induced alterations in IL-2r expression influence immune function.

Interferon

There is one report of an increase in IFNα after 1 hr cycling at 70% of $\dot{V}O_2$max (Viti, Muscettola, Paulesu, Bocci, & Almi, 1985). IFN activity, as measured by a plaque reduction assay on virally infected cells and compared to IFN standards, increased 100% immediately and 1 hr after exercise and returned to preexercise values by 2 hr

(Figure 6.2). The increased IFN activity was due to IFNα only, because it was heat-labile and inhibited by anti-IFNα neutralizing antibodies. The significance of transient increases in IFNα activity is uncertain at present. IFNα exhibits antiviral activity, stimulating cytotoxic cells and inhibiting viral replication (Roitt et al., 1989). An exercise-induced increase in IFNα may be related to increases in NK and macrophage activity noted after exercise (see chapters 4 and 7). However, as with the other cytokines discussed here, it is premature to draw conclusions from the limited literature. Exercise does not appear to change plasma levels of IFNγ (Haahr et al., in press; Viti et al.).

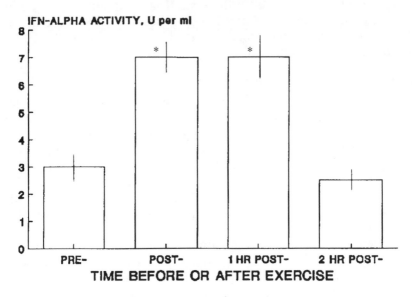

Figure 6.2 Plasma interferon after exercise. Interferon (IFN) activity was measured in plasma obtained before and after 1 hr of cycling at 70% V̇O₂max. IFN activity was titrated using a plaque reduction assay on virally infected cells, with titers expressed relative to reference standards. Bars represent SEM. *$p < .01$ compared to preexercise values.
Note. From "Effect of Exercise on Plasma Interferon Levels" by A. Viti, M. Muscettola, L. Paulesu, V. Bocci, and A. Almi, 1985, *Journal of Applied Physiology*, **59**, p. 427. Copyright 1985 by The American Physiological Society. Adapted by permission.

Interleukin-6

Plasma IL-6 concentration increases after prolonged exercise (Flegel et al., 1989; Haahr et al., in press) in parallel with an increase in

IL-1 level (Haahr et al.). For example, most (15 of 17) trained runners exhibited up to a 2-fold increase in IL-6 after a 42-km marathon; plasma IL-6 returned to baseline levels by 24 hr of recovery (Flegel et al.). IL-6 is one factor involved in the acute phase response to infection, and its release is stimulated by IL-1. It has been suggested that there is a coordinated release of IL-1, IL-6, and CRP during or after exercise, which may be related to muscle damage or a general inflammatory response (Espersen et al., 1990; Evans et al., 1986).

Tumor Necrosis Factor

There are only a few reports on the effects of exercise on TNF. When measured by enzyme-linked immunosorbent assay or bioassay, TNFα was not found in detectable levels either before or after a 42-km marathon (Flegel et al., 1989) or more moderate exercise, such as 1 hr of cycling at 75% $\dot{V}O_2$max (Haahr et al., in press). However, a more sensitive radioimmunoassay showed detectable levels in plasma from trained runners (Espersen et al., 1990). TNFα was unchanged immediately after but increased 2 hr after a 5-km race; normal levels were restored by 24 hr postrace (Espersen et al.). TNFα also appears to be elevated after moderate exercise (60 min at 60% $\dot{V}O_2$max) when measured with radioimmunoassay. However, at this work load only untrained individuals exhibit increases in TNFα level (Smith, Telford, Baker, et al., 1990). The increase in TNFα levels observed after exercise may be related to transitory increases in circulating monocyte number (Espersen et al.).

TNFα exhibits activities similar to IL-1, such as induction of the acute phase response, stimulation of monocyte antitumor activity, and B and T cell activation. In some instances IL-1 and TNFα act synergistically (Beutler & Cerami, 1990; Dinarello, 1990). Release of TNFα is stimulated by endotoxin, and naturally occurring levels of endotoxin appear to increase following intense prolonged exercise (Bosenberg, Brock-Utne, Gaffin, Wells, & Blake, 1988). It is unclear whether exercise-induced release of endotoxin and TNFα are related and whether transitory increases in TNFα influence the immune response.

Cytokine Synergism: A Role in Tissue Repair?

IL-1, IL-6, and TNFα have many similar and overlapping functions and may act synergistically; IL-1 and TNFα may stimulate the release of each other as well as IL-6 (reviewed by Dinarello, 1990, and Le & Vilcek, 1989). The effects of these cytokines are similar to many of the changes in immune and other physiological parameters observed with exercise, such as these (Dinarello):

- Increased body temperature (IL-1, IL-6, TNFα)
- Increased NK cytotoxic activity (IL-1, IL-6, TNFα)
- Macrophage activation (IL-1, IL-6, TNFα)
- Increased neutrophil oxidative activity (TNFα)
- Release of acute phase reactants (IL-1, IL-6, TNFα) and PGE (TNFα)
- Enhanced antibody production (IL-6)

Thus, it would not be unexpected if all three cytokines increase during exercise. However, the literature on this is sparse, and studies reporting increases in IL-1, IL-6, and TNFα have used widely different exercise protocols (Cannon et al., 1986; Flegel et al., 1989; Haahr et al., in press; Smith, Telford, Baker, et al., 1990). It remains to be seen if the three cytokines increase concomitantly under various exercise conditions, mediate the changes described, and influence immune function.

IL-1 and TNFα may also be involved in muscle degradation and repair following injury, as often occurs during intense activity. Both cytokines stimulate protein catabolism, fibroblast proliferation, and collagen synthesis (reviewed by Dinarello, 1990, and Piela & Korn, 1990) and are mediators of inflammation. However, an apparent lack of correlation between IL-1 and serum creatine kinase levels after exercise (Cannon et al., 1986) and between IL-6 and muscle soreness (K. Wooley, personal communication, 1991) suggest that there is no straightforward relationship between these cytokines and muscle damage or repair following exercise. Study on the relationship between the immune response and inflammatory/reparative processes resulting from exercise has only begun; it may be a fruitful area for future research.

Summary and Conclusions

Acute exercise appears to alter circulating levels of cytokines, such as IL-1, IL-2, IL-6, IFNα, and TNFα. IL-1, IL-6, and TNFα exhibit overlapping functions and may act synergistically. Exercise-induced increases in cytokines (IL-1, IFNα, TNFα) may be related to enhanced cytotoxic activity observed after exercise. It has also been suggested that changes in cytokines (IL-1, IL-6, TNFα) may reflect inflammation resulting from muscle degradation, and subsequent repair, following intense prolonged exercise. At present there are no reports on the effects of exercise on other cytokines, such as CSF, other interleukins, and TNFβ.

Levels of all cytokines studied to date appear to be within normal ranges even when elevated after exercise (Espersen et al., 1990). It is currently unclear whether exercise-induced changes in cytokines influence immune function. Biological activity of a particular cytokine depends upon its concentration, the cell type and environment, and levels of other cytokines; moreover, cytokines may behave differently in vivo compared to in vitro. It is difficult at this point to determine the effects on immune function of exercise-induced changes in a single cytokine.

Chapter 7

Exercise and Cytotoxic Cells

Cytotoxic (killing) activity is exhibited by several types of immune cells, in particular cytotoxic T lymphocytes (CTL), NK cells, and monocytes/macrophages. As described in chapter 2, CTL and NK cells are major effectors of host defense against tumor growth and virally infected cells.

Recent attention has focused on the effects of exercise on cytotoxic activity for several reasons: Exercise appears to influence host defense against both cancer and viral infections. Exercise also enhances circulating levels of cytokines involved in resistance to tumors and viral infection, such as IFN, TNF, IL-1, and IL-2. Moreover, stress influences resistance to tumor growth and viral infection, and some stress hormones modulate immune cell response to tumors; exercise also increases circulating stress hormone levels. Thus, it can be postulated that exercise may influence host defense against tumor growth and viral infection via modulating activity of cytotoxic cells. Most research in this area has focused on NK cells.

Exercise and NK Cells

NK cells are a distinct but heterogeneous subset of lymphocytes capable of recognizing and killing virally infected cells, certain tumor cells, and some microorganisms without prior exposure. The exact lineage of NK cells is still debated, but it is generally accepted that virtually all NK activity is mediated by large granular lymphocytes (LGL). NK activity and ADCC are mediated by the same cells.

The effect of exercise on NK cells has been recently reviewed (Mackinnon, 1989), although several papers have been published since. Total NK activity is generally increased during and immediately after exercise, whether brief or prolonged, moderate or intense (Berk et al., 1990; Brahmi et al., 1985; Deuster, Curiale, Cowan, & Finkelman, 1988; Edwards et al., 1984; Fiatarone et al., 1988; Kappel et al., in press; Kotani et al., 1987; Mackinnon et al., 1988;

Pedersen et al., 1988, 1989, 1990; Targan, Britvan, & Dorey, 1981; Watson et al., 1986).

For brief exercise (30 min or less), NK activity is restored to resting levels by 1 hr after exercise; in contrast, maximal or prolonged exercise may decrease total NK activity for 1 to 6 hr after cessation of exercise (Figures 7.1a and 7.1b) (Berk et al., 1990; Brahmi et al., 1985; Kappel et al., in press; Mackinnon et al., 1988; Pedersen et al., 1988). NK activity is also elevated by exercise in individuals over age 65 (Crist, Mackinnon, Thompson, Atterbom, & Egan, 1989; Fiatarone et al., 1989).

Resting NK Activity in Athletes

There has been one report of a decrease in resting NK activity following intense endurance exercise training in previously un-trained subjects (Watson et al., 1986). However, the percentage and number of circulating NK cells were not reported, and it is unclear whether the decrease in total NK activity represents lower cellular killing activity or changes in the relative proportions of lymphocytes (Mackinnon, 1989).

Resting and postexercise NK activity in athletes appear to be within the normal range (Brahmi et al., 1985; Mackinnon et al., 1988; Pedersen et al., 1989). Moreover, when compared between athletes and nonathletes, NK activity was similar or slightly elevated (by 25%) in athletes (Pedersen et al., 1989). In addition, both resting and postexercise NK activity were higher in women over age 65 who had undergone a moderate exercise program than in control women who had not exercise-trained (Crist et al., 1989). These data suggest that baseline NK activity is either unchanged or slightly increased by exercise training.

NK Subsets and Cytotoxic Activity

Total NK activity reflects both the killing activity of each cytotoxic cell and the number of cells in the assay system, and exercise may influence each parameter independently (Mackinnon, 1989). The assay system commonly used to measure total cytotoxic activity is an in vitro system with a mixture of lymphocytes, of which NK cells comprise about 15%. Any change in the relative proportion of lymphocyte subsets, such as occurs during exercise, may thus influence total cytotoxic activity. There is debate over the relation-ship between changes in lymphocyte subsets and NK cytotoxic activity during and after exercise (Berk et al., 1990; Mackinnon). In some instances, it appears that changes in circulating NK cell

glandins (PGE_1, PGE_2, PGA_1, PGA_2) are known inhibitors of NK cytotoxic activity, and PGE_2 production by monocytes increases after exercise (Pedersen et al., 1990).

In untrained individuals, 1 hr of cycling at 80% $\dot{V}O_2$max stimulated NK activity in cells obtained near the end of exercise. NK activity was suppressed in cells obtained 2 hr after exercise (Figure 7.2) (Kappel et al., 1991; Pedersen et al., 1988, 1990). Oral administration of the prostaglandin inhibitor indomethacin before exercise did not affect the increase in NK activity during exercise, but did prevent the decrease after (Pedersen et al., 1990).

Similar suppression of NK activity was noted when prostaglandins were added to cells in vitro (Kappel et al., in press). However, NK activity was normal when monocyte-depleted lymphocytes were used in the in vitro cytotoxic assay. Moroever, suppression of NK activity after exercise was related to an increase in monocyte number. These data suggest that a monocyte-derived factor, such as prostaglandins, is released after exercise and that this factor suppresses NK activity. The suppressive effect appears to be transitory, because NK activity is restored by 6 hr after intense prolonged exercise (Berk et al., 1990).

Catecholamines

Exercise-induced changes in NK activity and cell distribution are similar to those induced by administration of epinephrine in physiological doses. For example, NK activity increased 40% during 1 hr of moderate cycling and then decreased 30% below preexercise levels 2 hr after exercise (Kappel et al., 1991). Similar changes in NK activity were noted with infusion of epinephrine at doses that increased plasma epinephrine concentration to the level observed during exercise. Exercise and epinephrine infusion induced similar changes in CD16 (NK) cell number (i.e., higher during exercise and normal by 2 hr postexercise). These data indicate that epinephrine mediates at least part of the change in NK cell distribution and cytotoxic activity during and after exercise.

Exercise and Other Cytotoxic Cells

ADCC occurs by a somewhat different mechanism than does NK cytotoxicity, although both activities are mediated by the same cell, the NK cell or LGL. It is not unexpected, therefore, that exercise-induced changes in ADCC are similar to those observed for NK cells (Hanson & Flaherty, 1981; Hedfors et al., 1978). ADCC increases by

20% to 40% early in exercise (Hedfors et al., 1978) and remains elevated during exercise lasting 1 hr (Hanson & Flaherty). The number of cells exhibiting ADCC increases at the same time as killing activity; however, the magnitude of increase in cell number is larger than for killing activity (Hanson & Flaherty), suggesting that inactive cells may be recruited into the circulation during exercise.

Although cytotoxic T lymphocytes (CTL) are important effectors in cell-mediated cytotoxicity against tumor and virally infected cells, there do not appear to be any reports on the effects of exercise on CTL activity.

Summary and Conclusions

There appears to be a dual effect of exercise on NK activity. Total cytotoxic activity increases during both submaximal and maximal exercise. This increase appears to be related to selective recruitment of NK cells into the circulation early in exercise and possibly to stimulation of killing activity by soluble factors released during exercise. These factors include epinephrine and, possibly, IL-1, IFNα, TNFα, and β-endorphin. There may be a synergistic effect of these factors in augmenting NK activity during exercise.

In contrast, NK activity is suppressed from 1 to 2 hr after maximal or prolonged exercise. This suppression may be due to a decreased number of circulating NK cells as well as to suppression of killing activity by factors such as prostaglandins. The prostaglandin-induced suppression of NK activity after exercise appears to be due to an increase in circulating monocyte number and a concomitant rise in plasma prostaglandin concentration. After prolonged exercise, total NK activity is restored toward normal before NK cell number (6 vs. 21 hr, respectively) (Berk et al., 1990), suggesting that suppression of killing is transitory. Restoration of cytotoxic activity despite low NK cell number several hours after exercise may indicate (1) increased killing by each cell, (2) recruitment of a more active cell, (3) activation of previously inactive cells, or (4) a combination of effects.

Chapter 8

Clinical Implications of Exercise

One reason for the growing interest in exercise and immune function is the possible clinical implications: Might exercise play a role in the prevention and treatment of certain illnesses, such as cancer or acquired immune deficiency syndrome (AIDS)? Epidemiological evidence indicates an association between regular physical activity and lower incidence of certain cancers. Animal studies also suggest that exercise training enhances resistance to experimentally induced tumor growth. In addition, exercise is now being used in treatment of diseases like cancer and AIDS, primarily to maintain or improve functional capacity and to counteract some of the debilitating physical effects of disease or treatment. For example, regular exercise may help maintain muscle strength and flexibility in cancer patients, many of whom experience muscle weakness as a result of treatment. Regular exercise may also have positive psychological effects, improving general psychological state in patients faced with life-threatening disease or undergoing uncomfortable treatment.

That physical activity may also have positive effects on the immune system is implicit in current research in this area. If positive effects can be shown, then exercise may have a role in stimulating the immune system during times of illness or reduced responsiveness (e.g., aging or AIDS). It is also possible that a lifetime of regular exercise may maintain the immune system at its optimum, perhaps preventing illness.

Exercise and Cancer

The topic of exercise and cancer has been reviewed several times in recent years (Bartram & Wynder, 1989; Eichner, 1987b; Gauthier, 1986; Kohl, LaPorte, & Blair, 1988; Shephard, 1986). Several recent epidemiological studies over extended periods (10-20 years) have reported reduced incidence of cancer in physically active groups (Albanes, Blair, & Taylor, 1989; Blair et al., 1989; Paffenbarger,

Hyde, & Wing, 1987). For example, a major cohort study showed a significant relationship between self-reported physical activity and cancer risk at all sites in both men and women (Albanes et al.). Relative risk was 80% higher in inactive compared to moderately active men; it was 30% higher in inactive compared to active women. Differences in risk could not be attributed to factors such as cigarette smoking or body mass.

There is also strong evidence that occupational physical activity is associated with a reduced risk of colorectal cancer. Relative risk of colon cancer is elevated between 1.3 and 2 times in inactive compared to more active groups (Ballard-Barbash et al., 1990; Garabrant, Peters, Mack, & Bernstein, 1984; Peters, Garabrant, Yu, & Mack, 1989; Seversson, Nomura, Grove, & Stemmerman, 1989; Vena et al., 1985; Wu, Paganini-Hill, Ross, & Henderson, 1987).

Physical activity may also reduce the risk of cancer at other sites, such as the breast and reproductive system in women (Albanes et al., 1989; Frisch et al., 1985; Vena, Graham, Zielezny, Brasure, & Swanson, 1987). For example, in a retrospective study of 5,400 college alumnae, the incidences of breast and reproductive system cancer were consistently lower in former athletes compared to non-athletes (Figures 8.1a and 8.1b; Frisch et al., 1985). Because proportionately more former athletes remained physically active than did nonathletes (74% vs. 57%, respectively), it is possible that continued activity was related to the lower incidence of cancer. Although the effects of exercise on cancer at other cites has not been studied extensively, there are also reports of reduced incidence of cancer of the lung (Albanes et al., 1989; Seversson et al., 1989) and of the thyroid and the digestive and hematopoietic systems (Frisch, Wyshak, Albright, Albright, & Schiff, 1989) in active groups. Physical activity does not appear to be related to cancer of the skin (Frisch et al., 1989).

Mechanisms Influencing the Relationship Between Exercise and Cancer

A variety of mechanisms have been proposed to explain an association between physical activity and cancer risk in humans (Bartram & Wynder, 1989; Eichner, 1987b; Kohl et al., 1988). Exercise may influence cancer risk by reducing body fat and the incidence of obesity; obesity is considered a risk factor for certain cancers, including endometrial, breast, and colon cancer. Exercise may also influence the level of certain hormones, such as estradiol, which is considered a causative agent in some forms of breast cancer.

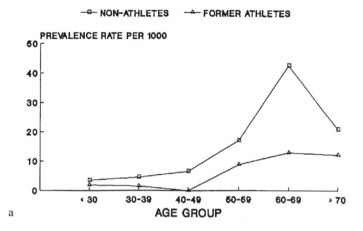

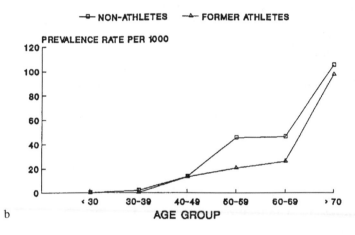

Figure 8.1   Prevalence rates of cancers of the reproductive system (a) and breast (b) of former athletes and nonathletes. Age-specific rates of prevalence for cancer of the reproductive system (uterus, ovary, cervix, vagina) and breast were determined in 5,398 female alumnae (classes 1925 to 1981) of universities and colleges. The women were classified as either former athletes (during college; n = 2,622) or nonathletes (n = 2,776).
Note. From "Lower Prevalence of Breast Cancer and Cancers of the Reproductive System Among Former College Athletes Compared to Non-Athletes" by R.E. Frisch, G. Wyshak, N.L. Albright, T.E. Albright, I. Schiff, K.P. Jones, J. Witschi, E. Shiang, E. Koff, and M. Marguglio, 1985, *British Journal of Cancer*, **52**, pp. 887-888. Copyright 1985 by Macmillan Press. Adapted by permission.

Individuals who choose to exercise or to work in physically demanding occupations may be more likely to adopt healthier lifestyles, thus reducing risk of cancer associated with such factors as smoking and high-fat diets. Regular physical activity may reduce stress levels, which may have a positive effect on resistance to cancer, or may augment the immune system's defense against tumor growth. Finally, some common genetic factors may predispose an individual to both physical activity and low risk of cancer.

Animal Studies

Experimental animal models have several advantages over human models for studying the effects of exercise on tumor growth, including a shorter duration and control of possible confounding factors such as body mass and the amount of exercise performed. Animal models may also provide unique information about the mechanisms underlying exercise-induced modulation of tumor resistance.

With one exception (Thompson, Ronan, Ritacco, & Tagliafero, 1989), animal studies over nearly 50 years have shown that exercise inhibits growth of a variety of experimentally induced tumors (Andrianopoulus, Nelson, Bombeck, & Souza, 1987; Cohen, Choi, & Wang, 1988; Good & Fernandes, 1981; Hoffman, Paschkis, DeBias, Cantarow, & Williams, 1962; Rashkis, 1952; Rusch & Kline, 1944). In virtually all studies showing reduced tumor growth, animals began exercise days or weeks before introduction of tumors and continued exercise after. For example, in mice that had been swim-trained before and then 2 weeks after tumor implantation, survival time was increased by 20% compared to untrained mice with the same tumor (Rashkis, 1952). When training was discontinued 14 days after implantation, tumor growth was greatly accelerated in formerly trained mice, eventually equaling that in the control group. These data suggest that any inhibitory effect of exercise on tumor growth persists only as long as training is maintained.

Exercise appears to influence resistance to tumor growth via a complex interaction of dietary factors, body composition, and possibly immune factors. However, changes in body composition or diet cannot fully account for the effects of exercise on tumor growth (Cohen et al., 1988; Hoffman et al., 1962; Thompson et al., 1989). Energy restriction and low-fat diets may enhance both resistance to tumor growth and activity of cytotoxic cells (Hebert, Barone, Reddy, & Blacklund, 1990). An early report suggested that exercise may cause release of soluble factors that enhance resistance to tumor growth (Hoffman et al.).

Exercise in the Treatment of Cancer

Cancer patients may exhibit training effects after moderate exercise programs (MacVicar & Winningham, 1986; MacVicar, Winningham, & Nickel, 1989). For example, $\dot{V}O_2$max increased 40% in Stage II breast cancer patients on chemotherapy after exercise training (cycling at 60% to 85% $\dot{V}O_2$max, 20 to 30 min, 3 times per week for 10 weeks). There was a concomitant improvement in mood state, as measured by the Profile of Mood States (POMS), with a significant reduction in total mood disturbance in the exercisers; during the same time nonexercised patients exhibited an increase in total mood disturbance (MacVicar & Winningham).

Exercised patients also maintained body weight and fat compared with nonexercised patients, who increased body weight and fat (normal during chemotherapy for breast cancer) (Winningham, Mac-Vicar, Bondoc, Anderson, & Minton, 1989). A surprising finding was that the exercised patients also reported reduced nausea during the training period (MacVicar & Winningham, 1986). These data suggest that moderate exercise may improve functional capacity and mood state in cancer patients while possibly counteracting some of the negative effects of treatment. The authors noted that these were limited data on a single type of cancer and that further work is needed to determine whether moderate exercise has positive effects in other cancer patients.

Guidelines for exercise in cancer patients were put forward by the same authors (Winningham, MacVicar, & Burke, 1986), who emphasized an individualized approach for exercise prescription. Some cancers or treatments may interfere with adaptation to training, such as by decreasing protein synthesis. Moreover, symptoms or the effects of illness or treatment (e.g., nausea, weakness) may limit the ability to exercise regularly. It is important to consider specific drugs used in therapy, because some are associated with cardiac or pulmonary myopathies or arythmias (Stone, Copelan, Weisbrode, & Rozmiarek, 1986). It was recommended that cancer patients not exercise on the same day as chemotherapy (Winningham et al., 1986). Finally, it was noted that exercise may be inappropriate for some cancer patients or at certain stages of the disease.

Exercise in the Treatment of AIDS

Acquired immune deficiency syndrome, first recognized in Western medicine in the late 1970s, is caused by the human immunodeficiency virus–Type I (HIV-1). HIV-1 gains entry into T lymphocytes via binding to the CD4 receptor on T_H cells; once infected, T_H cells die. Marked reductions in circulating T_H cell number and in the ratio of T_H to T_S cells are the hallmarks of HIV infection. Because activation of the T_H cell is essential in initiating the immune response, deficiency of T_H cells results in abnormal responses of many aspects of immune function. Deficiency of T_H cells subsequently leaves the body vulnerable to a variety of opportunistic diseases.

It has been suggested that behavioral interventions, such as exercise, stress management, and relaxation, may help restore immunocompetence in HIV-1–infected patients, especially in early stages of infection (Antoni et al., 1990; LaPerriere, Schneiderman, Antoni, & Fletcher, 1990). These authors (LaPerriere, Schneiderman, Antoni, & Fletcher, 1990) presented a model in which stressors (mood states and social stressors) alter levels of stress hormones that adversely influence the immune response to the virus. It was reasoned that physical and psychological interventions may alter the neuroendocrine responses to stressors and improve mood state, improving immune responsiveness during early stages of infection. For example, exercise training may decrease anxiety and depression, leading to release of endogenous opioids or reduced release of corticosteroids, either or both of which may enhance immune function (LaPerriere, Schneiderman, et al., 1990).

As part of a larger intervention project, HIV-1 seropositive asymptomatic men participated in an aerobic training program (45 min cycling at 80% age-predicted maximum heart rate, 3 times per week for 10 weeks) (Antoni et al., 1990; LaPerriere, Schneiderman, et al., 1990). A group of seropositive men who did not exercise were control subjects; groups of noninfected (seronegative) men also were included for comparison. $\dot{V}O_2max$ increased after training in both infected and noninfected exercised men. Both groups also exhibited increases in the number of CD4 cells (specifically the CD4 subset involved in activation of CD8 cells) and in mature B cells, although responses were of lesser magnitude in infected than in noninfected exercisers. In contrast, nonexercised seropositive men exhibited no changes in CD4 or B cell numbers.

NK cell number was also maintained after notification of antibody (infected) status in HIV-1 positive men who had undergone prior exercise training (HIV+ EX in Figure 8.2); in contrast, HIV-1 positive men who had not exercised (HIV+ C) exhibited marked reductions in NK cell number upon notification of infected status (Figure 8.2) (LaPerriere, Antoni, et al., 1990). Because NK cells are important in defense against viral infection, maintenance of NK cell number by

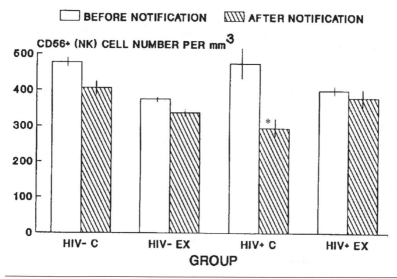

Figure 8.2   Natural killer cell number after exercise training in HIV-1 positive men. NK cell (CD56+ or NKH-1+) number was assessed by flow cytometry. Cells were obtained from HIV-positive or -negative men 72 hr before and 1 week after notification of serological status (HIV antibody positive or negative). Exercised men had undergone 5 weeks of aerobic exercise training (see text); control men had not exercised during this time. Abbreviations: HIV– = HIV negative; HIV+ = HIV positive; C = control subjects; EX = exercise trained subjects. Bars represent SEM. *$p <$ .05 compared to before notification.

Note. From "Exercise Intervention Attenuates Emotional Distress and Natural Killer Cell Decrements Following Notification of Positive Serological Status for HIV-1" by A.R. Laperriere, M.H. Antoni, N. Schneiderman, G. Ironson, N. Klimas, P. Caralis, and M.A. Fletcher, 1990, *Biofeedback and Self-Regulation,* **15**, p. 238. Copyright 1990 by Plenum Publishing Corporation. Adapted by permission.

exercise may enhance defense against HIV-1 as well as opportunistic infections.

Seropositive exercisers also exhibited no change in tension/anxiety, as measured by POMS 72 hr after they were informed of an infection diagnosis, compared to seropositive control subjects who showed marked increase in tension/anxiety at the same time (Antoni et al., 1990). These limited data suggest that regular aerobic exercise may enhance both immunological and psychological responses during early HIV-1 infection, before symptoms appear, and especially upon notification of antibody status, a time of great stress for high-risk persons.

It has been noted that exercise testing and prescription for the HIV-1 patient must be individualized. Exercise capacity may be limited in those who are HIV-1 positive, even when they show no obvious signs of illness. For example, it has been reported that asymptomatic HIV-1 positive men exhibit abnormal cardiorespiratory responses to standard exercise testing; changes included reduced aerobic exercise capacity, mild tachypnea, lower ventilatory threshold, and increased slope of the heart rate to $\dot{V}O_2$ relationship (Johnson et al., 1990). It was suggested that these changes may be indicative of subclinical cardiac abnormalities associated with HIV-1 infection.

Summary and Conclusions

Regular physical activity appears to reduce the incidence of cancer in humans and to enhance resistance to tumor growth in experimental animal models, suggesting a possible role of exercise in long-term prevention of cancer. Moderate exercise is also recommended as adjunct therapy in some illnesses, such as cancer and AIDS, primarily to counteract the debilitating effects of disease and treatment and to enhance the patient's psychological state. Recent data also suggest that moderate exercise may enhance immune function in early HIV-1 infection. At present, it is unclear whether the immunomodulating effects of exercise occur directly via action on immune function or indirectly via alterations in other parameters, such as psychological stress and neuroendocrine factors. The long-term effects of exercise on immune function in patients with disease have not been thoroughly explored.

Chapter 9

Exercise and Immunology: Present and Future Directions

Having reviewed current literature describing the effects of exercise on various aspects of immune function and having touched on the complexities of the immune system, I want to summarize what is known and then look to the future.

Table 9.1 summarizes our state of knowledge on the effects of exercise on immune parameters; I have categorized the effects as potentially positive, negative, or neutral (no effect). Four major points are apparent:

1. Exercise alters many aspects of immune function, in both positive and negative directions; some immune parameters are unaffected by exercise.
2. Exercise influences the immune response at the level of the intact organism (e.g., survival during infections) as well as individual immune parameters (e.g., lymphocyte proliferation).
3. Response of a specific immune function varies with exercise intensity and individual fitness level.
4. There are inconsistencies in the immune response to exercise that cannot yet be fully explained (e.g., both increased and decreased specific antibody responses).

Models to Explain Mechanisms Underlying the Immune Response to Exercise

In the several models put forward to explain possible mechanisms underlying the response of particular immune parameters to exercise, the common theme is the role of neuroendocrine factors. Many hormones capable of immunomodulation are released during

Table 9.1   Potentially Positive, Negative, and Neutral Effects of Exercise on Immune Parameters

Potentially positive	Potentially negative
Resistance to illness	
↑Survival in viral infection[a]	↑Incidence of URI[b]
↑Survival in bacterial infection[a]	↑Paralysis with polio[b,d]
↓Incidence of cancer[a]	↓Survival in viral infection[d]
Leukocyte distribution	
Recruitment into circulation	↓T_H: T_S ratio
Lymphocyte proliferation	
↑B cell response[a]	↓T cell response[b]
Innate immunity	
↑Neutrophil killing	↓Neutrophil killing[c]
↑Macrophage activity	↓Macrophage killing[b]
↑Acute phase proteins	↓Complement[c]
Humoral immunity	
↑Specific antibody response[a,e]	↓Specific antibody response[b,c]
	Delayed antibody response[d]
	↓Mucosal IgA[b,c]
Cytokines	
↑IL-1, IL-6, TNFα, IFNα	↓Resting IL-1 level[c]
	↓IL-2 concentration
	↓IL-2 receptor number
Cytotoxicity	
↑NK killing	↓NK activity 2 hr postexercise[b]
↑ADCC killing	
↑Macrophage cytostatic activity	

Neutral (no effect)
Resting leukocyte number[c]
Serum Ig
Lymphocyte proliferation[e]
Mucosal IgA[e]
Macrophage cytotoxic activity

Note. Data were compiled from various sources.

[a]Only with prior exercise training. [b]Only during and after intense exercise. [c]In athletes compared to nonathletes. [d]Only with exercise at time of infection. [e]Only during and after moderate exercise.

exercise, such as epinephrine, ACTH, cortisol, β-endorphin, met-enkephalin, prolactin, growth hormone, and thyroxine. Moreover, regular exercise (i.e., training) changes the response of several of these hormones to exercise, usually by blunting exercise-induced release, which may account for training-induced changes or differences between athletes and nonathletes in the immune response to exercise.

Figure 9.1 is one example of a model recently proposed to explain the apparent dual response of neutrophils to exercise (Smith & Weidemann, 1990). The diagram shows how moderate exercise may induce priming of neutrophil microbicidal capacity through immunostimulatory pituitary hormones and/or an endotoxin-monokine cascade. These mechanisms may work synergistically or independently. Priming may be negated, however, by very intensive exercise, due to activation of the immunosuppressive arm of the pituitary-adrenal axis. The initial switch may be triggered by local hypothalamic/pituitary factors once exercise intensity reaches a critical threshold level. Immunosuppression may be manifested as a consequence of sustained ACTH and cortisol release caused by high concentrations of monokines. Although this model was developed to explain a particular immune response (neutrophil microbicidal activity), many features may be generalized to other immune parameters. For example, growth hormone, IL-1, and TNF also enhance other immune parameters, such as NK cytotoxicity. The model addresses the complex interaction of neuroendocrine factors (e.g., hormones) and cytokines, as well as both stimulatory and inhibitory effects of some hormones. Moreover, the model attempts to explain why moderate exercise appears to stimulate immune function, whereas intense or prolonged exercise often results in immunosuppression.

Briefly, Smith and Weidemann propose that moderate exercise increases release of immunostimulatory hormones, such as growth hormone, prolactin, and β-endorphin, as well as cytokines such as IL-1 and TNF. On the other hand, intense exercise is associated with dramatic increases in circulating catecholamines and corticosteroids, which inhibit a number of immune parameters. This model is also consistent with the observation that most instances of reduced immune reactivity occur in elite athletes during intense training and major competition, a time of psychological and physical stress.

Although several models have been proposed to explain specific immune responses to exercise, research on exercise and immunology is not yet at the stage where a single model can fully explain the complex interactions of the physiological responses to exercise and

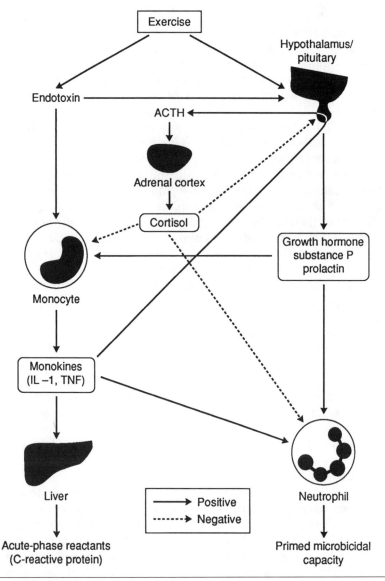

Figure 9.1 Proposed relationship between neuroendocrine and immune changes during exercise. This model, or parts of it, may also be applicable to other aspects of immune function besides neutrophil activity.

Note. From "The Exercise and Immunity Paradox: A Neuroendocrine/Cytokine Hypothesis" by J.A. Smith and M.J. Weidemann, 1990, *Medical Science Research*, **18**, p. 751. Copyright 1990 by Science and Technology Letters. Reproduced by permission of Science and Technology Letters.

how these may influence immune function. For example, some hormones exhibit dual effects on immune parameters, depending on dosage, time of exposure, and the nature of exposure (e.g., in vivo vs. in vitro administration). Clearly, further research is needed to elucidate the mechanisms by which exercise influences immune function. It is likely that several schemes may be necessary to fully explain the immune response to exercise.

Future Directions

The field of exercise and immunology is still in its infancy, particularly with regard to understanding the effect of exercise on resistance to disease and the mechanisms responsible for exercise-induced changes in immune function. I have briefly outlined several possible directions for research that may further our understanding.

1. The general perception that athletes are more susceptible to certain illnesses (e.g., URI, mononucleosis) during intense training and major competition has yet to be clearly established by objective study. It is important to determine whether athletes are indeed at risk and, if so, to identify aspects of training (e.g., specific sport, exercise intensity or duration, and adequacy of recovery) and competition (e.g., psychological stress) that are related to susceptibility to illness. A cross-disciplinary approach using knowledge from exercise physiology, immunology, clinical medicine, sport psychology, and coaching would greatly enhance our understanding of how exercise influences resistance to illness among athletes.

2. Most studies on the effects of exercise on immune function have focused on short-term changes following a single bout of exercise or short-term training. The long-term effects of regular exercise training have received relatively little attention. The potential long-term effects of exercise on immune function have obvious implications for health promotion and preventive medicine, especially in nations with increasingly active and expanding older populations.

3. Early studies on exercise and immune function made many intriguing observations that have yet to be fully explored. For example, early work on animal models noted that prior exercise training enhances resistance to experimental illness, whereas exercise introduced at the time of infection impairs resistance to infection. With a few exceptions, this apparent dual nature of the immune response to exercise has not been addressed in any systematic way, nor have the responsible mechanisms been elucidated. Research in this area

may also add to the growing body of literature on regulation of immune function.

4. As described in chapter 8, exercise is now being used as adjunct therapy in some diseases, such as cancer and AIDS. With the prime motivation being to enhance "quality of life," only a few research groups are studying the immune response to exercise among these patients. Early data suggest that exercise may beneficially alter immune function; for example, circulating T_H (CD4) cell number increases after exercise training in HIV-1–positive men. At present, it is unclear whether exercise influences immune function directly or indirectly (e.g., by reducing psychological stress) in these patients. Exercise is one mode of therapy for psychological disorders, such as depression, which have also been associated with immunosuppression. The potential role of exercise in abrogating the negative effects of physical and psychological stress has implications for clinical medicine as well as basic research in immunology.

Finally, research has just begun to address the mechanisms responsible for exercise-induced changes in immune function. Future applications of technology in immunology and molecular biology to research on the immune response to exercise will greatly enhance our understanding of the body's response to exercise as well as regulation of the immune system.

Glossary

acquired immunity—"Adaptive" immunity involving antibody and immune cell responses specific to the infectious agent. Acquired immunity results in "memory," preventing later disease by the same agent.

ADCC (antibody-dependent cell-mediated cytotoxicity)—Cytotoxic activity by large granular lymphocytes that recognize certain antibodies on the target cell.

aerobic exercise—Endurance-type exercise, lasting up to hours (e.g., distance running or cycling), that relies on oxidative metabolism as the major source of energy production.

antibody—An immunoglobulin molecule that can bind specifically to a particular antigen.

antigen—A protein that induces an antibody response.

antigen presenting cells—Diverse cell types able to present antigen on their cell surface and thus stimulate immune cells.

APP/APR (acute phase proteins or reactants)—A heterogeneous class of serum glycoproteins that increase in concentration during inflammation and infection.

B cell—A type of lymphocyte capable of producing antibody. B cells differentiate into plasma cells.

bactericidal—Able to kill bacteria.

CD (cluster designation)—Cell surface proteins, identified with monoclonal antibodies, that are used to classify different types of leukocytes.

complement—A group of 20 serum proteins involved in inflammation and humoral immunity.

ConA (concanavalin A)—A substance that stimulates T cell proliferation.

CRP (C-reactive protein)—An acute phase protein found in serum during inflammation and infection.

CSF (colony-stimulating factors)—A group of cytokines that stimulate hematopoietic stem cell proliferation and differentiation.

CTL, T_c (cytotoxic T lymphocyte)—A subset of T cell capable of killing certain tumor and virally infected cells.

cytokine—A soluble factor produced by myriad cells involved in communication between immune cells. Many cytokines are growth factors.

cytostatic—Able to inhibit cellular growth.

cytotoxic—Able to kill cells.

eccentric exercise—Movement in which a muscle generates tension while lengthening. Eccentric exercise occurs mainly in stabilizing the body against gravity and is associated with muscle fiber damage and delayed muscle soreness.

granulocyte—A heterogeneous class of leukocytes characterized by a multilobed nucleus and intracellular granules. Granulocytes are comprised of neutrophils, eosinophils, basophils, and mast cells.

granulocytosis—Increase in circulating granulocyte number.

humoral immunity—Immune function via soluble factors found in blood and other body fluids.

IFN (interferon)—A class of unrelated cytokines with antiviral activity and the capacity to stimulate certain immune cells.

Ig (immunoglobulin)—Glycoprotein found in blood and other body fluids that may exert antibody activity. All antibodies are Ig molecules, but not all Ig exhibit antibody activity.

IL (interleukin)—A class of unrelated cytokines involved in communication between immune cells. At least 12 interleukin molecules have been identified.

IL-2r (interleukin 2 receptor)—Receptor for IL-2 found on activated lymphocytes.

isometric—Static muscle contraction in which the muscle generates tension but does not change length.

leukocyte—Heterogeneous cells found in the circulation and various tissues with diverse functions related to the immune response.

leukocytosis—Increase in circulating leukocyte number.

LPS (lipopolysaccharide)—A substance that stimulates B cell proliferation.

lymphocyte—Mononuclear immune cell.

lymphocytosis—Increase in circulating lymphocyte number.

macrophage—A phagocytic cell residing in tissues and derived from the monocyte.

maximum heart rate (age-predicted)—Highest possible heart rate, usually achieved during maximal exercise. Maximum heart rate decreases with age and can be estimated as 220 – age.

mitogen—A substance that stimulates cell division (mitosis) in lymphocytes.

monocyte—A circulating phagocytic leukocyte, which can differentiate into a macrophage upon migration into tissue.

mucosal immunity—Immune function related to the body's external surfaces of the gut and the oro-nasal, respiratory, and genitourinary tracts.

neutrophil—A phagocytic leukocyte characterized by a multilobed nucleus and many intracellular granules.

NK (natural killer) cell—A large granular lymphocyte capable of killing certain tumor and virally infected cells.

PHA (phytohemmaglutinin)—A substance that stimulates T cell proliferation.

phagocytosis—A process by which a leukocyte (monocyte, neutrophil) engulfs, ingests, and degrades a foreign particle or organism.

plasma cell—Mature antibody-secreting cell derived from the B cell.

PWM (pokeweed mitogen)—A substance that stimulates T cell–dependent B cell proliferation.

T cell (lymphocyte)—A heterogeneous population of lymphocytes comprising helper/inducer T cells and cytotoxic/suppressor T cells.

T_H (helper T lymphocyte)—A subset of T lymphocyte capable of recognizing antigen and producing several lymphokines that activate other immune cells.

TNF (tumor necrosis factor)—A cytokine with many actions, such as antiviral and antitumor activity, increasing body temperature, and activating certain immune cells.

T_S (suppressor T lymphocyte)—A subset of T lymphocyte capable of suppressing activity of other immune cells or processes.

URI (upper respiratory illness)—Infectious illness involving the oral and nasal regions (e.g., cold, sore throat).

$\dot{V}O_2max$—Maximum oxygen consumption, usually expressed as a volume of oxygen consumed per minute. $\dot{V}O_2max$ is used as an indicator of maximal exercise power and to standardize exercise rate between individuals (e.g., exercising at 60% of one's $\dot{V}O_2max$).

References

Ahlborg, B., & Ahlborg, G. (1970). Exercise leukocytosis with and without beta-adrenergic blockade. *Acta Medica Scandinavica,* **187**, 241-246.

Albanes, D., Blair, A., & Taylor, P.R. (1989). Physical activity and risk of cancer in the NHANES I population. *American Journal of Public Health,* **79**, 744-750.

Andrianopoulus, G., Nelson, R.L., Bombeck, C.T., & Souza, G. (1987). The influence of physical activity in 1,2 dimethylhydrazine induced colon carcinogenesis in the rat. *Anticancer Research,* **7**, 849-852.

Antoni, M.H., Schneiderman, N., Fletcher, M.A., Goldstein, D.A., Ironson, G., & LaPerriere, A. (1990). Psychoneuroimmunology and HIV-1. *Journal of Consulting and Clinical Psychology,* **58**, 38-49.

Bailey, G.H. (1925). The effect of fatigue upon the susceptibility of rabbits to intratracheal injections of type I pneumococcus. *American Journal of Hygiene,* **5**, 175-295.

Ballard-Barbash, R., Schatzkin, A., Albanes, D., Schiffman, M.H., Kreger, B.E., Kannel, W.B., Anderson, K.M., & Helsel, W.E. (1990). Physical activity and risk of large bowel cancer in the Framingham study. *Cancer Research,* **50**, 3610-3613.

Bartram, H.P., & Wynder, E.L. (1989). Physical activity and colon cancer risk? Physiological considerations. *The American Journal of Gastroenterology,* **84**, 109-112.

Berglund, B., & Hemmingsson, P. (1990). Infectious disease in elite cross-country skiers: A one-year incidence study. *Clinical Sports Medicine,* **2**, 19-23.

Berk, L.S., Nieman, D.C., Youngberg, W.S., Arabatzis, K., Simpson-Westerberg, M., Lee, J.W., Tan, S.A., & Eby, W.C. (1990). The effect of long endurance running on natural killer cells in marathoners. *Medicine and Science in Sports and Exercise,* **22**, 207-212.

Beutler, B., & Cerami, A. (1990). Cachectin (tumor necrosis factor) and lymphotoxin as primary mediators of tissue catabolism, inflammation, and shock. In S. Cohen (Ed.), *Lymphokines and the immune response* (pp. 199-211). Boca Raton, FL: CRC Press.

Bieger, W.P., Weiss, M., Michel, G., & Weicker, H. (1980). Exercise-induced monocytosis and modulation of monocyte function. *International Journal of Sports Medicine*, **1**, 30-36.

Blair, S.N., Kohl, H.W., Paffenbarger, R.S., Clark, D.G., Cooper, K.H., & Gibbons, L.W. (1989). Physical fitness and all-cause mortality: A prospective study of healthy men and women. *Journal of the American Medical Association*, **262**, 2395-2401.

Blecha, R., & Minocha, H.C. (1983). Suppressed lymphocyte blasto-genic responses and enhanced *in vitro* growth of infectious bovine rhinotracheitis virus in stressed feeder calves. *American Journal of Veterinary Research*, **44**, 2145-2148.

Bosenberg, A.T., Brock-Utne, J.G., Gaffin, S.L., Wells, M.T.B., & Blake, G.T.W. (1988). Strenuous exercise causes systemic endo-toxemia. *Journal of Applied Physiology*, **65**, 106-108.

Brahmi, Z., Thomas, J.E., Park, M., Park, M., & Dowdeswell, I.R.G. (1985). The effect of acute exercise on natural killer-cell activity of trained and sedentary human subjects. *Journal of Clinical Immunology*, **5**, 321-328.

Brooks, G.A., & Fahey, T.D. (1985). *Exercise physiology: Human bioenergetics and its applications*. New York: Macmillan.

Busse, W.W., Anderson, C.L., Hanson, P.G., & Folts, J.D. (1980). The effect of exercise on the granulocyte response to isoproterenol in the trained athlete and unconditioned individual. *Journal of Allergy and Clinical Immunology*, **65**, 358-364.

Cabinian, A.E., Kiel, R.J., Smith, F., Ho, K.L., Khatib, R., & Reyes, M.P. (1990). Modification of exercise-aggravated coxsackievirus B3 murine myocarditis by T lymphocyte suppression in an inbred model. *Journal of Laboratory and Clinical Medicine*, **115**, 454-462.

Cannon, J.G., Evans, W.J., Hughes, V.A., Meredith, C.N., & Dina-rello, C.A. (1986). Physiological mechanisms contributing to increased interleukin-1 secretion. *Journal of Applied Physiology*, **61**, 1869-1874.

Cannon, J.G., & Kluger, M.J. (1983). Endogenous pyrogen activity in human plasma after exercise. *Science*, **220**, 617-619.

Cannon, J.G., & Kluger, M.J. (1984). Exercise enhances survival rate in mice infected with *Salmonella typhimurium. Proceedings of the Society for Experimental Biology and Medicine*, **175**, 518-521.

Christensen, R.D., & Hill, H.H. (1987). Exercise-induced changes in the blood concentration of leukocyte populations in teenage athletes. *The American Journal of Pediatric Hematology/Oncology*, **9**, 140-142.

Cohen, L.A., Choi, K., & Wang, C.-X. (1988). Influence of dietary fat, caloric restriction, and voluntary exercise on N-nitrosomethyl-urea-induced mammary tumorigenesis in rats. *Cancer Research*, **48**, 4276-4283.

Cohen, S. (Ed.) (1990). *Lymphokines and the immune response.* Boca Raton, FL: CRC Press.

Cowles, W.N. (1918). Fatigue as a contributory cause of pneumonias. *Boston Medical and Surgery Journal*, **179**, 555.

Crist, D.M., Mackinnon, L.T., Thompson, R.F., Atterbom, H.A., & Egan, P.A. (1989). Physical exercise increases natural cellular-mediated tumor cytotoxicity in elderly women. *Gerontology*, **35**, 66-71.

Daniels, W.L., Sharp, D.S., Wright, J.E., Vogel, J.A., Friman, G., Beisel, W.R., & Knapik, J.J. (1985). Effects of virus infection on physical performance in man. *Military Medicine*, **150**, 1-8.

Davidson, R.J.L., Robertson, J.D., Galea, G., & Maughan, R.J. (1987). Hematological changes associated with marathon running. *International Journal of Sports Medicine*, **8**, 19-25.

Deuster, P.A., Curiale, A.M., Cowan, M.L., & Finkelman, F.D. (1988). Exercise-induced changes in populations of peripheral blood mononuclear cells. *Medicine and Science in Sports and Exercise*, **20**, 276-280.

Dinarello, C.A. (1990). Interleukin-1 and its biologically related cytokines. In S. Cohen (Ed.), *Lymphokines and the immune response* (pp. 145-179). Boca Raton, FL: CRC Press.

Douglas, D.J., & Hanson, P.G. (1978). Upper respiratory infections in the conditioned athlete. *Medicine and Science in Sport*, **10**, 55.

Dufaux, B., & Order, U. (1989). Complement activation after prolonged exercise. *Clinica Chimica Acta*, **179**, 45-50.

Dufaux, B., Order, U., Geyer, H., & Hollmann, W. (1984). C-reactive protein serum concentration in well-trained athletes. *International Journal of Sports Medicine*, **5**, 102-106.

Eberhardt, A. (1971). Influence of motor activity on some serologic mechanisms of nonspecific immunity of the organism. *Acta Physiologica Polonica*, **22**, 185-194.

Edwards, A.J., Bacon, T.H., Elms, C.A., Verardi, R., Felder, M., & Knight, S.C. (1984). Changes in the populations of lymphoid cells in human peripheral blood following physical exercise. *Clinical Experimental Immunology*, **58**, 420-427.

Eichner, E.R. (1987a). Infectious mononucleosis: Recognition and management in athletes. *The Physician and Sportsmedicine*, **15**, 61-70.

Eichner, E.R. (1987b). Exercise, lymphokines, calories, and cancer. *The Physician and Sportsmedicine*, **15**, 109-116.

Eskola, J., Ruuskanen, O., Soppi, E., Viljanen, M.K., Jarvinen, M., Toivonen, H., & Kouvalainen, K. (1978). Effect of sport stress on lymphocyte transformation and antibody formation. *Clinical Experimental Immunology, 32*, 339-345.

Espersen, G.T., Elbaek, A., Ernst, E., Toft, E., Kaalund, S., Jersild, C., & Grunnet, N. (1990). Effect of physical exercise on cytokines and lymphocyte subpopulations in human peripheral blood. *APMIS, 98*, 395-400.

Evans, W.J., Meredith, C.N., Cannon, J.G., Dinarello, C.A., Frontera, W.R., Hughes, V.A., Jones, B.H., & Knuttgen, H.G. (1986). Metabolic changes following eccentric exercise in trained and untrained men. *Journal of Applied Physiology, 61*, 1864-1868.

Fehr, H.-G., Lotzerich, H., & Michna, H. (1989). Human macrophage function and physical exercise: Phagocytic and histochemical studies. *European Journal of Applied Physiology, 58*, 613-617.

Ferry, A., Picard, F., Duvallet, A., Weill, B., & Rieu, M. (1990). Changes in blood leucocyte populations induced by acute maximal and chronic submaximal exercise. *European Journal of Applied Physiology, 59*, 435-442.

Fiatarone, M.A., Morley, J.E., Bloom, E.T., Benton, D., Makinodan, T., & Solomon, G.F. (1988). Endogenous opioids and the exercise-induced augmentation of natural killer cell activity. *Journal of Clinical Laboratory Medicine, 112*, 544-552.

Fiatarone, M.A., Morley, J.E., Bloom, E.T., Benton, D., Solomon, G.F., & Makinodan, T. (1989). The effect of exercise on natural killer cell activity in young and old subjects. *Journal of Gerontology, 44*, M37-45.

Flegel, W.A., Mannel, D.N., Baumstark, M., Berg, A., & Northoff, H. (1989). Serum levels of monokines (IL1, TNFα, and IL6) in long-distance runners. In *Abstracts of the Seventh International Congress of Immunology* (p. 447). Stuttgart, Germany: Gustav Fischer Verlag.

Foster, C., Pollock, M., Farrell, P., Maksud, M., Anholm, J., & Hare, J. (1982). Training responses of speed skaters during a competitive season. *Research Quarterly for Exercise and Sport, 53*, 243-246.

Foster, N.K., Martyn, J.B., Rangno, R.E., Hogg, J.C., & Pardy, R.L. (1986). Leukocytosis of exercise: Role of cardiac output and catecholamines. *Journal of Applied Physiology, 61*, 2218-2223.

Friman, G. (1977). Effect of acute infectious disease on isometric muscle strength. *Scandinavian Journal of Clinical Laboratory Investigation, 37*, 303-308.

Frisch, R.E., Wyshak, G., Albright, N.L., Albright, T.E., & Schiff, I. (1989). Lower prevalence of non-reproductive system cancers among female former college athletes. *Medicine and Science in Sports and Exercise,* **21**, 250-253.

Frisch, R.E., Wyshak, G., Albright, N.L., Albright, T.E., Schiff, I., Jones, K.P., Witschi, J., Shiang, E., Koff, E., & Marguglio, M. (1985). Lower prevalence of breast cancer and cancers of the reproductive system among former college athletes compared to non-athletes. *British Journal of Cancer,* **52**, 885-891.

Galun, E., Burstein, R., Assia, E., Tur-Kaspa, I., Rosenblum, J., & Epstein, Y. (1987). Changes of white blood cell count during prolonged exercise. *International Journal of Sports Medicine,* **8**, 253-255.

Garabrant, D.H., Peters, J.M., Mack, T.M., & Bernstein, L. (1984). Job activity and colon cancer risk. *American Journal of Epidemiology,* **119**, 1105-1114.

Gatmaitan, B.G., Chason, J.L., & Lerner, A.M. (1970). Augmentation of the virulence of murine coxsackie-virus B-3 myocardiopathy by exercise. *Journal of Experimental Medicine,* **131**, 1121-1136.

Gauthier, M.M. (1986). Can exercise reduce the risk of cancer? *The Physician and Sportsmedicine,* **14**, 171-178.

Gimenez, M., Mohan-Kumar, T., Humbert, J.C., de Talance, N., & Buisine, J. (1986). Leukocyte, lymphocyte and platelet response to dynamic exercise: Duration or intensity effect? *European Journal of Applied Physiology,* **55**, 465-470.

Gimenez, M., Mohan-Kumar, T., Humbert, J.C., de Talance, N., Teboul, M., & Belenguer, F.J.A. (1987). Training and leucocyte, lymphocyte and platelet response to dynamic exercise. *Journal of Sports Medicine,* **27**, 172-177.

Gmunder, F.K., Lorenzi, G., Bechler, B., Joller, P., Muller, J., Ziegler, W.H., & Cogoli, A. (1988). Effect of long-term physical exercise on lymphocyte reactivity: Similarity to spaceflight reactions. *Aviation, Space, and Environmental Medicine,* **59**, 146-151.

Good, R.A., & Fernandes, G. (1981). Enhancement of immunologic function and resistance to tumor growth in Balb/c mice by exercise. *Federation Proceedings,* **40**, 1040.

Graham, N.M.H., Douglas, R.M., & Ryan, P. (1986). Stress and acute respiratory infection. *American Journal of Epidemiology,* **124**, 389-401.

Green, R.L., Kaplan, S.S., Rabin, B.S., Stanitski, C.L., & Zdziarski, U. (1981). Immune function in marathon runners. *Annals of Allergy,* **47**, 73-75.

Haahr, P.M., Pedersen, B.K., Fomsgaard, A., Tvede, N., Diamant, M., Klarlund, K., Halkjaer-Kristensen, J., & Bendtzen, K. (in press). Effect of physical exercise on *in vitro* production of interleukin 1, interleukin 6, tumour necrosis factorα, interleukin 2, and interferonα. *International Journal of Sports Medicine.*

Hamblin, A.S. (1988). *Lymphokines.* Oxford: IRL Press.

Hanson, P.G., & Flaherty, D.K. (1981). Immunological responses to training in conditioned runners. *Clinical Science,* **60,** 225-228.

Hebert, J.R., Barone, J., Reddy, M.M., & Backlund, J.-Y.C. (1990). Natural killer cell activity in a longitudinal dietary fat intervention trial. *Clinical Immunology and Immunopathology,* **54,** 103-116.

Hedfors, E., Biberfeld, P., & Wahren, J. (1978). Mobilization to the blood of human non-T and K lymphocytes during physical exercise. *Journal of Clinical Laboratory Immunology,* **1,** 159-162.

Hedfors, E., Holm, G., Ivansen, M., & Wahren, J. (1983). Physiological variation of blood lymphocyte reactivity: T-cell subsets, immunoglobulin production, and mixed-lymphocyte reactivity. *Clinical Immunology and Immunopathology,* **27,** 9-14.

Hedfors, E., Holm, G., & Ohnell, B. (1976). Variations of blood lymphocytes during work studied by cell surface markers, DNA synthesis and cytotoxicity. *Clinical Experimental Immunology,* **24,** 328-335.

Hoffman, S.A., Paschkis, K.E., DeBias, D.A., Cantarow, A., & Williams, T.L. (1962). The influence of exercise on the growth of transplanted rat tumors. *Cancer Research,* **22,** 597-599.

Hoffman-Goetz, L., Keir, R., Thorne, M.E., & Houston, C. (1986). Chronic exercise in mice depresses splenic T lymphocyte mitogenesis in vitro. *Clinical Experimental Immunology,* **66,** 551-557.

Hoffman-Goetz, L., Thorne, R.J., & Houston, M.E. (1988). Splenic immune responses following treadmill exercise in mice. *Canadian Journal of Physiology and Pharmacology,* **66,** 1415-1419.

Hoffman-Goetz, L., Thorne, R., Randall-Simpson, J.A., & Arumugam, Y. (1989). Exercise stress alters murine lymphocyte subset distribution in spleen, lymph nodes and thymus. *Clinical Experimental Immunology,* **76,** 307-310.

Horstmann, D.M. (1950). Acute poliomyelitis: Relation of physical activity at the time of onset to the course of the disease. *Journal of the American Medical Associaion,* **142,** 236-241.

Ilback, N.-G., Fohlman, J., & Friman, G. (1989). Exercise in coxsackie B3 myocarditis: Effects on heart lymphocyte subpopulations and the inflammatory reaction. *American Heart Journal,* **117,** 1298-1302.

Ilback, N.-G., Friman, G., Beisel, W.R., Johnson, A.J., & Berendt, R.F. (1984). Modifying effects of exercise on clinical course and biochemical response of the myocardium in influenza and tularemia in mice. *Infection and Immunity,* **45**, 498-504.

Jemmott, J.B., Borysenko, M., Chapman, R., Borysenko, J.Z., McClelland, D.C., Meyer, D., & Benson, H. (1983). Academic stress, power motivation, and decrease in secretion rate of salivary secretory immunoglobulin A. *Lancet,* **1**, 1400-1402.

Johnson, J.E., Anders, G.T., Blanton, H.M., Hawkes, C.E., Bush, B.A., McAllister, C.K., & Matthews, J.I. (1990). Exercise dysfunction in patients seropositive for the human immunodeficiency virus. *American Review of Respiratory Diseases,* **141**, 618-622.

Kappel, M., Tvede, N., Galbo, H., Haahr, P.M., Kjaer, M., Linstouw, M., Klarlund, K., & Pedersen, B.K. (in press). Evidence that the effect of physical exercise on natural killer cell activity is mediated by adrenaline. *Journal of Applied Physiology.*

Kassil, G.N., Levando, V.A., Suzdal'nitskii, R.S., Pershin, B.B., & Kuz'min, S.N. (1988). Neuro-humoral regulation of immune homeostasis during adaptation to extreme stresses using modern sport as a model. *Sports Training, Medicine and Rehabilitation,* **1**, 61-65.

Kiel, R.J., Smith, F.F., Chason, J., Khatib, R., & Reyes, M.P. (1989). Coxsackievirus B3 myocarditis in C3H/HeJ mice: Description of an inbred model and the effect of exercise on virulence. *European Journal of Epidemiology,* **5**, 348-350.

Kohl, H.W., LaPorte, R.E., & Blair, S.N. (1988). Physical activity and cancer: An epidemiological perspective. *Sports Medicine,* **6**, 222-237.

Kotani, T., Aratake, Y., Ishiguro, R., Yamamoto, I., Uemura, Y., Tamura, K., & Ohtaki, S. (1987). Influence of physical exercise on large granular lymphocytes, Leu-7 bearing mononuclear cells and natural killer activity in peripheral blood—NK-cell and NK-activity after physical exercise. *Acta Haematologica Japonica,* **50**, 1210-1216.

Lanier, L.L., Le, A.M., Civin, C.I., Loken, M.R., & Phillips, J.H. (1986). The relationship of CD16 (Leu-11) and Leu-19 (NKH-1) antigen expression on human peripheral blood NK cells and cytototoxic T lymphocytes. *The Journal of Immunology,* **136**, 4480-4486.

LaPerriere, A.R., Antoni, M.H., Schneiderman, N., Ironson, G., Klimas, N., Caralis, P., & Fletcher, M.A. (1990). Exercise intervention attenuates emotional distress and natural killer cell decrements following notification of positive serologic status for HIV-1. *Biofeedback and Self-Regulation,* **15**, 229-242.

LaPerriere, A., Schneiderman, H., Antoni, M.H., & Fletcher, M.A. (1990). Aerobic exercise training and psychoneuroimmunology in AIDS research. In A. Baum & L. Temoshok (Eds.), *Psychological Aspects of AIDS* (pp. 259-286). Hillsdale, NJ: Erlbaum.

Le, J., & Vilcek, J. (1989). Interleukin 6: A multifunctional cytokine regulating immune reactions and the acute phase protein response. *Laboratory Investigation*, **61**, 588-602.

Levando, V.A., Suzdal'nitskii, R.S., Pershin, B.B., & Zykov, M.P. (1988). Study of secretory and antiviral immunity in sportsmen. *Sports Training, Medicine and Rehabilitation*, **1**, 49-52.

Levinson, S.O., Milzer, A., & Lewin, P. (1945). Effect of fatigue, chilling and mechanical trauma on resistance to experimental poliomyelitis. *American Journal of Hygiene*, **42**, 204-213.

Lewicki, R., Tchorzewski, H., Denys, A., Kowalska, M., & Golinska, A. (1987). Effect of physical exercise on some parameters of immunity in conditioned sportsmen. *International Journal of Sports Medicine*, **8**, 309-314.

Lewicki, R., Tchorzewski, H., Majewska, E., Nowak, Z., & Baj, Z. (1988). Effect of maximal physical exercise on T-lymphocyte subpopulations and on interleukin 1 (IL 1) and interleukin 2 (IL 2) production *in vitro*. *International Journal of Sports Medicine*, **9**, 114-117.

Liesen, H., Dufaux, B., & Hollmann, W. (1977). Modifications of serum glycoproteins the days following a prolonged physical exercise and the influence of physical training. *European Journal of Applied Physiology*, **37**, 243-254.

Liu, Y.G., & Wang, S.Y. (1986/87). The enhancing effect of exercise on the production of antibody to *Salmonella typhi* in mice. *Immunology Letters*, **14**, 117-120.

Lotzerich, H., Fehr, H.-G., & Appell, H.-J. (1990). Potentiation of cytostatic but not cytolytic activity of murine macrophages after running stress. *International Journal of Sports Medicine*, **11**, 61-65.

Mackinnon, L.T. (1989). Exercise and natural killer cells: What is the relationship? *Sports Medicine*, **7**, 141-149.

Mackinnon, L.T., Chick, T.W., van As, A., & Tomasi, T.B. (1988). Effects of prolonged intense exercise on natural killer cell number and function. In C.O. Dotson & J.H. Humphrey (Eds.), *Exercise physiology: Current selected research*, Vol. 3 (pp. 77-89). New York: AMS Press.

Mackinnon, L.T., Chick, T.W., van As, A., & Tomasi, T.B. (1989). Decreased secretory immunoglobulins following intense endurance exercise. *Sports Training, Medicine, and Rehabilitation*, **1**, 209-218.

Mackinnon, L.T., Ginn, E., & Seymour, G. (1990). Comparison of the effects of exercise during training and competition on secretory IgA levels. *Medicine and Science in Sports and Exercise*, **22**, S125.

Mackinnon, L.T., Ginn, E., & Seymour, G. (1991). Temporal relationship between exercise-induced decreases in salivary IgA concentration and subsequent appearance of upper respiratory illness in elite athletes. *Medicine and Science in Sports and Exercise*, **23**, S45.

Mackinnon, L.T., Ginn, E., & Seymour, G. (in press). Effects of exercise during sports training and competition on salivary IgA levels. *Behaviour and Immunity Proceedings of the 1990 Australian Behavioural Immunology Group Scientific Meeting*. Boca Raton, FL: CRC Press.

MacVicar, M.G., & Winningham, M.L. (1986). Promoting the functional capacity of cancer patients. *The Cancer Bulletin*, **38**, 235-239.

MacVicar, M.G., Winningham, M.L., & Nickel, J.L. (1989). Effects of aerobic interval training on cancer patients' functional capacity. *Nursing Research*, **38**, 348-351.

Mahan, M.P., & Young, M.R. (1989). Immune parameters of untrained or exercise-trained rats after exhaustive exercise. *Journal of Applied Physiology*, **66**, 282-287.

McCarthy, D.A., & Dale, M.M. (1988). The leucocytosis of exercise: A review and model. *Sports Medicine*, **6**, 333-363.

Moorthy, A.V., & Zimmerman, S.W. (1978). Human leukocyte response to an endurance race. *European Journal of Applied Physiology*, **38**, 271-276.

Muir, A.L., Cruz, A., Martin, B.A., Thommasen, H., Belzberg, A., & Hogg, J.C. (1984). Leukocyte kinetics in the human lung: Role of exercise and catecholamines. *Journal of Applied Physiology*, **57**, 711-719.

Muns, G., Liesen, H., Riedel, H., & Bergmann, K.-Ch. (1989). Influence of long-distance running of IgA in nasal secretion and saliva. *Deutsche Zeitschrift für Sportmedizin*, **40**, 63-65.

Nehlsen-Cannarella, S.L., Nieman, D.C., Balk-Lamberton, A.J., Markoff, P.A., Chritton, D.B.W., Gusewitch, G., & Lee, J.W. (1991). The effect of moderate exercise training on immune response. *Medicine and Science in Sports and Exercise*, **23**, 64-70.

Nicholls, E.E., & Spaeth, R.A. (1922). The relation between fatigue and the susceptibility of guinea pigs to infections of type I pneumococcus. *American Journal of Hygiene*, **2**, 527-535.

Nieman, D.C., Berk, L.S., Simpson-Westerberg, M., Arabatzis, K., Youngberg, S., Tan, S.A., Lee, J.W., & Eby, W.C. (1989). Effects of long-endurance running on immune system parameters and lymphocyte function in experienced marathoners. *International Journal of Sports Medicine*, **10**, 317-323.

Nieman, D.C., Johanssen, L.M., & Lee, J.W. (1989). Infectious episodes in runners before and after a roadrace. *The Journal of Sports Medicine and Physical Fitness*, **29**, 289-296.

Nieman, D.C., Johanssen, L.M., Lee, J.W., & Arabatzis, K. (1990). Infectious episodes in runners before and after the Los Angeles Marathon. *Journal of Sports Medicine and Physical Fitness*, **30**, 316-328.

Nieman, D.C., Tan, S.A., Lee, J.W., & Berk, L.S. (1989). Complement and immunoglobulin levels in athletes and sedentary controls. *International Journal of Sports Medicine*, **10**, 124-128.

Oppenheimer, E.H., & Spaeth, R.A. (1922). The relation between fatigue and the susceptibility of rats towards a toxin and an infection. *American Journal of Hygiene*, **2**, 51-66.

Oshida, Y., Yamanouchi, K., Hayamizu, S., & Sato, Y. (1988). Effect of acute physical exercise on lymphocyte subpopulations in trained and untrained subjects. *International Journal of Sports Medicine*, **9**, 137-140.

Paffenbarger, R.S., Hyde, R.T., & Wing, A.L. (1987). Physical activity and incidence of cancer in diverse populations: A preliminary report. *American Journal of Clinical Nutrition*, **45**, 312-317.

Pahlavani, M.A., Cheung, T.H., Chesky, J.A., & Richardson, A. (1988). Influence of exercise on the immune function of rats of various ages. *Journal of Applied Physiology*, **64**, 1997-2001.

Pedersen, B.K., Tvede, N., Christensen, L.D., Klarlund, K., Kragbak, S., & Halkjaer-Kristensen, J. (1989). Natural killer cell activity in peripheral blood of highly trained and untrained persons. *International Journal of Sports Medicine*, **10**, 129-131.

Pedersen, B.K., Tvede, N., Hansen, F.R., Andersen, V., Bendix, T., Bendixen, G., Bendtzen, K., Galbo, H., Haahr, P.M., Klarlund, K., Sylvest, J., Thomsen, B.S., & Halkjaer-Kristensen, J. (1988). Modulation of natural killer cell activity in peripheral blood by physical exercise. *Scandinavian Journal of Immunology*, **27**, 673-678.

Pedersen, B.K., Tvede, N., Klarlund, K., Christensen, L.D., Hansen, F.R., Galbo, H., & Kharazmi, A. (1990). Indomethacin *in vitro* and *in vivo* abolishes post-exercise suppression of natural killer cell activity in peripheral blood. *International Journal of Sports Medicine*, **11**, 127-131.

Pershin, B.B., Kuz'min, S.N., Suzdal'nitskii, R.S., & Levando, V.A. (1988). Reserve potential of immunity. *Sports Training, Medicine and Rehabilitation,* **1**, 53-60.

Peters, E.M., & Bateman, E.D. (1983). Ultramarathon running and upper respiratory tract infections. *South African Medical Journal,* **64**, 582-584.

Peters, R.K., Garabrant, D.H., Yu, M.C., & Mack, T.M. (1989). A case-control study of occupational and dietary factors in colorectal cancer in young men by subsite. *Cancer Research,* **49**, 5459-5468.

Piela, T.H., & Korn, J.H. (1990). Lymphokines and cytokines in the reparative process. In S. Cohen (Ed.), *Lymphokines and the immune response* (pp. 256-273). Boca Raton, FL: CRC Press.

Priest, J.B., Oei, T.O., & Moorehead, W.R. (1982). Exercise-induced changes in common laboratory tests. *American Journal of Clinical Pathology,* **77**, 285-289.

Rashkis, H.A. (1952). Systemic stress as an inhibitor of experimental tumors in Swiss mice. *Science,* **116**, 169-171.

Reyes, M.P., & Lerner, A.M. (1976). Interferon and neutralizing antibody in sera of exercised mice with coxsackievirus B-3 myocarditis. *Proceedings of the Society for Experimental Biology and Medicine,* **151**, 333-338.

Ricken, K.-H., Rieder, T., Hauck, G., & Kindermann, W. (1990). Changes in lymphocyte subpopulations after prolonged exercise. *International Journal of Sports Medicine,* **11**, 132-135.

Roberts, J.A. (1985). Loss of form in young athletes due to viral infection. *British Medical Journal,* **290**, 357-358.

Roberts, J.A. (1986). Viral illnesses and sports performance. *Sports Medicine,* **3**, 296-303.

Robertson, A.J., Ramesar, K.C.R.B., Potts, R.C., Gibbs, J.H., Browning, M.C.K., Brown, R.A., Hayes, P.C., & Beck, J.S. (1981). The effect of strenuous physical exercise on circulating blood lymphocytes and serum cortisol levels. *Journal of Clinical Laboratory Immunology,* **5**, 53-57.

Roitt, I., Brostoff, J., & Male, D. (1989). *Immunology.* London: Gower Medical.

Rose, R.J., & Bloomberg, M.S. (1989). Response to sprint exercise in the greyhound: Effects on haematology, serum biochemistry and muscle metabolites. *Research in Veterinary Science,* **47**, 212-218.

Rosenbaum, H.E., & Harford, C.G. (1953). Effects of fatigue on susceptibility of mice to poliomyelitis. *Proceedings of the Society for Experimental Biology and Medicine,* **83**, 678-681.

Round, J.M., Jones, D.A., & Cambridge, G. (1987). Cellular infiltrates in human skeletal muscle: Exercise induced damage as a model for inflammatory muscle disease? *Journal of the Neurological Sciences, 82*, 1-11.

Rusch, H.P., & Kline, B.E. (1944). The effect of exercise on the growth of a mouse tumor. *Cancer Research, 4*, 116-118.

Sawka, M.N., Young, A.J., Dennis, R.C., Gonzalez, R.R., Pandolf, K.B., & Valeri, C.R. (1989). Human intravascular immunoglobulin response to exercise-heat and hypohydration. *Aviation, Space, and Environmental Medicine, 60*, 634-638.

Schaefer, R.M., Kokot, K., Heidland, A., & Plass, R. (1987). Joggers' leukocytes. *The New England Journal of Medicine, 316*, 223-224.

Seversson, R.K., Nomura, A.M.Y., Grove, J.S., & Stemmermann, G.N. (1989). A prospective analysis of physical activity and cancer. *American Journal of Epidemiology, 130*, 522-529.

Shephard, R.J. (1986). Exercise and malignancy. *Sports Medicine, 3*, 235-241.

Simon, H.B. (1987). Exercise and infection. *The Physician and Sportsmedicine, 15*, 135-141.

Simpson, J.A.R., Hoffman-Goetz, L., Thorne, R., & Arumugam, Y. (1989). Exercise stress alters the percentage of splenic lymphocyte subsets in response to mitogen but not in response to interleukin-1. *Brain, Behavior, and Immunology, 3*, 119-128.

Smith, J.A., Telford, R.D., Baker, M.S., Hapel, A.J., & Weidemann, M.J. (1990). Moderate exercise increases plasma monokine but not lymphokine activity in men. *Blood , 76*, (suppl. 1), 194a.

Smith, J.A., Telford, R.D., Mason, I.B., & Weidemann, M.J. (1990). Exercise, training and neutrophil microbicidal activity. *International Journal of Sports Medicine, 11*, 179-187.

Smith, J.A., & Weidemann, M.J. (1990). The exercise and immunity paradox: A neuroendocrine/cytokine hypothesis. *Medical Science Research, 18*, 749-753.

Smith, L.L., McCammon, M., Smith, S., Chamness, M., Israel, R.G., & O'Brien, K.F. (1989). White blood cell response to uphill walking and downhill jogging at similar metabolic loads. *European Journal of Applied Physiology, 58*, 833-837.

Soppi, E., Varjo, P., Eskola, J., & Laitinen, L.A. (1982). Effect of strenuous physical stress on circulating lymphocyte number and function before and after training. *Journal of Clinical Laboratory Immunology, 8*, 43-46.

Steel, C.M., Evans, J., & Smith, M.A. (1974). Physiological variation in circulating B cell:T cell ratio in man. *Nature, 247*, 387-389.

Stites, D.P. (1987). Clinical laboratory methods for detection of cellular immune function. In D.P. Stites, J.D. Stobo, & J.V. Wells, (Eds.), *Basic and clinical immunology* (pp. 285-303). Norwalk, CT: Appleton & Lange.

Stone, D.W., Copelan, E.A., Weisbrode, S.E., & Rozmiarek, H. (1986). Effects of exercise on bleomycin-induced pulmonary toxicity in mice. *Cancer Treatment Reports*, **70**, 1067-1071.

Targan, S., Britvan, L., & Dorey, F. (1981). Activation of human NKCC by moderate exercise: Increased frequency of NK cells with enhanced capability of effector-target lytic interactions. *Clinical Experimental Immunology*, **45**, 352-360.

Tharp, G.D., & Barnes, M.W. (1990). Reduction of saliva immunoglobulin levels by swim training. *European Journal of Applied Physiology*, **60**, 61-64.

Thompson, H.J., Ronan, A.M., Ritacco, K.A., & Tagliafero, A.R. (1989). Effect of type and amount of dietary fat on the enhancement of rat mammary tumorigenesis by exercise. *Cancer Research*, **49**, 1904-1908.

Tomasi, T.B., & Plaut, A.G. (1985). Humoral aspects of mucosal immunity. In J.I. Gallin & A.S. Fauci (Eds.), *Advances in host defense mechanisms* (pp. 31-61). New Yor,k: Raven Press.

Tomasi, T.B., Trudeau, F.B., Czerwinski, D., & Erredge, S. (1982). Immune parameters in athletes before and after strenuous exercise. *Journal of Clinical Immunology*, **2**, 173-178.

Tvede, N., Pedersen, B.K., Hansen, F.R., Bendix, T., Christensen, L.D., Galbo, H., & Halkjaer-Kristensen, J. (1989). Effect of physical exercise on blood mononuclear cell subpopulations and in vitro proliferative responses. *Scandinavian Journal of Immunology*, **29**, 383-389.

Vena, J.E., Graham, S., Zielezny, M., Brasure, J., & Swanson, M.K. (1987). Occupational exercise and risk of cancer. *American Journal of Clinical Nutrition*, **45**, 318-327.

Vena, J.E., Graham, S., Zielezny, M., Swanson, M.K., Barnes, R.E., & Nolan, J. (1985). Lifetime occupational exercise and colon cancer. *American Journal of Epidemiology*, **122**, 357-365.

Viti, A., Muscettola, M., Paulesu, L., Bocci, V., & Almi, A. (1985). Effect of exercise on plasma interferon levels. *Journal of Applied Physiology*, **59**, 426-428.

Watson, R.R., Moriguchi, S., Jackson, J.C., Werner, L., Wilmore, J.H., & Freund, B.J. (1986). Modification of cellular immune function in humans by endurance exercise training during β-adrenergic blockade with atenolol or propranolol. *Medicine and Science in Sports and Exercise*, **18**, 95-100.

Wells, C.L., Stern, J.R., & Hecht, L.H. (1982). Hematological changes following a marathon race in male and female runners. *European Journal of Applied Physiology, 48*, 41-49.

Winningham, M.L., MacVicar, M.G., Bondoc, M., Anderson, J.I., & Minton, J.P. (1989). Effect of aerobic exercise on body weight and composition in patients with breast cancer on adjuvant chemotherapy. *Oncology Nursing Forum, 16*, 683-689.

Winningham, M.L., MacVicar, M.G., & Burke, C.A. (1986). Exercise for cancer patients: Guidelines and precautions. *The Physician and Sportsmedicine, 14*, 125-134.

Wit, B. (1984). Immunological response of regularly trained athletes. *Biology of Sport, 1*, 221-235.

Wong, D.W., Thompson, H.L., Thong, Y.H., & Thornton, J.R. (1990). Effect of strenuous exercise stress on chemiluminescence response of alveolar macrophages. *Equine Veterinary Journal, 22*, 33-35.

Woodruff, J.F. (1980). Viral myocarditis: A review. *American Journal of Pathology, 101*, 427-479.

Wu, A.H., Paganini-Hill, A., Ross, R.K., & Henderson, B.E. (1987). Alcohol, physical activity and other risk factors for colorectal cancer: A prospective study. *British Journal of Cancer, 55*, 687-694.

Index

About the Author

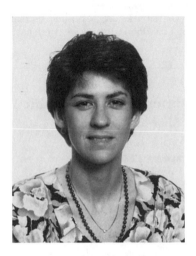

Dr. Laurel Traeger Mackinnon has over 10 years' experience in exercise science. Her current research includes a project funded by the Australian Sports Commission that explores immune response to training and overtraining in elite athletes.

Dr. Mackinnon earned her PhD in exercise science at the University of Michigan. She is senior lecturer in exercise physiology and exercise management at the University of Queensland in Brisbane, Queensland, Australia. She previously held the position of research assistant professor at the University of New Mexico School of Medicine.

Dr. Mackinnon is a fellow of the American College of Sports Medicine (ACSM) and a member of the Australian Sports Medicine Federation, the Australian Alliance for Physical Activity and Lifestyle, and the Australian Association of Health Promotion Professionals.

Human Kinetics Publishers

Current Issues in Exercise Science Series

Current Issues in Exercise Science is a series of monographs, each reporting on a hot topic of interest in exercise science. Written by leading scholars, these 80- to 144-page paperbacks are published quickly so the information is news, not history. A new title in the series is released every 3 to 4 months.

New Dimensions in Aerobic Fitness

Brian J. Sharkey, PhD

[Monograph Number 1]
1991 • Paper • 112 pp
Item BSHA0326 • ISBN 0-87322-326-8

How well does $\dot{V}O_2$max measure aerobic fitness? Is it the best measure of change in exercise prescription studies? Exercise physiologist Brian Sharkey examines these questions in *New Dimensions in Aerobic Fitness*, the first monograph in the Current Issues in Exercise Science series. The book challenges current thinking about the relevance and validity of this important measure and presents new ideas for measuring aerobic fitness.

Forthcoming issues in the CIES series

New Developments in Body Composition
Timothy G. Lohman, PhD

Exercise and Mental Health
Larry M. Leith, PhD

Exercise Endocrinology
Victoria J. Harber, PhD, and John R. Sutton, MD

 Human Kinetics Books
A Division of Human Kinetics Publishers, Inc.

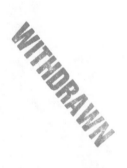